Intimacy On The Plate

Extra Trim Edition

**209 APHRODISIAC RECIPES TO SPICE UP
YOUR LOVE LIFE AT HOME TONIGHT**

Olga Petrenko

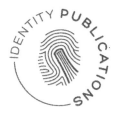

Intimacy On The Plate/Olga Petrenko —2nd ed.

ISBN-10: 1-945884-38-X

ISBN-13: 978-1-945884-38-2

Identity Publications

www.IdentityPublications.com

**To inquire about getting your own book or course produced,
published, or promoted, please send an email to:**
contact@identitypublications.com

Ordering Information:

Special discounts are available on quantity purchases by corpora-
tions, associations, and others at the web address above.

Intimacy On The Plate Original Edition is available at:
www.IntimacyOnThePlate.com

Contents

"Sharing food with another human being is an intimate act that should not be indulged in lightly."

– *M.F.K. Fisher*

Preface to the Extra Trim Edition

In February 2017, I saw my name and recipes appear in a real, professionally produced cookbook, selling on Amazon and other retailers. *Intimacy On The Plate* was the culmination of a lifetime of experimentation in the kitchen (and the bedroom), combined with the determination to see it all come together in a format that could be shared around the world. The finished product (available on Amazon or at www.intimacyontheplate.com) was a beautiful 8.5" square book, containing 316 full-color pages in a visual layout that captured the eye and invited the imagination. It was a book any cook could be proud to display on their shelf and that I felt proud to be the creator of.

As a first-time author, I was understandably nervous and indecisive when making the critical decisions about how the final product would come together and the launch would be organized. I had no reason for readers to take me seriously or assume my work would be any good. I knew the polished visual presentation would be an important part of convincing them to risk their money and their time on purchasing what I had put together. I have to thank my daughter, Anastasia, for being bold enough to insist that we go to print with the erogenous oyster design that ended up on the final cover, as it has received endless intrigue and praise, and I would have been far more reserved had it been left up to me what the cover should look like. The visual presentation was likely the single biggest factor in the book's early success. I'm so proud that we were able to bring together such a gorgeous table piece. *Intimacy On The Plate* was a hit, almost immediately becoming a bestseller in multiple Amazon categories, and even reaching the top 100 of all books on Amazon for a time.

Amidst the positive reception, with stories of readers using recipes from the book to stoke the fires of their intimacy arriving in my and my publisher's inbox, two recurring oversights became clear with the production and distribution of *Intimacy On The Plate*. First, the cost of printing a full-color book of this size was becoming too high to be able to offer the hardcover version of the book at a price that was within the range of what consumers were accustomed to paying for cookbooks. Second, many early buyers expressed that they loved the information and recipes, but found the large, thick size inconvenient for casual use ("that's what she said"). They wanted to be able to flip through the book more easily and scan the many recipes quickly and find a new one to try. They wanted to be able to throw it in a purse and show to a friend for a dinner date. And so, I realized it would be a worthwhile endeavor to prepare a new version of the book that offered the convenience readers were looking for, even at the cost of removing the gorgeous color photography and interior design I loved so much about the original edition. I would also be able to offer my beloved work at a more manageable price for those who just wanted the information and didn't necessarily care about the aesthetics of the design.

With a complete overhaul of the formatting and some light edits to the content (such as the inclusion of an index of ingredients), the *Extra Trim Edition* you are now reading was born. I hope you take the opportunity to share the love and wisdom contained here with those you care about. Bring it with you on your weekly shopping trip to get inspired erotic meal ideas from the ingredients available where you are. Share recipes with your friends who cook and come up with interesting ways to add to and customize the arrangements I've provided. Bring it with you on a romantic trip with your sweetheart and create an intimate mood on the go. Whether a drink, a snack, or a full-course meal, romantic moments that enhance our ability to show our physical love to the people we care about should be happening all the time, anywhere we are. That is my wish for you with the birth of this new edition, which is the product of a lifetime of love and research!

Many fans have reached out to me to ask how they can support the success of *Intimacy On The Plate* and spread the word of this unique, yet traditional approach to love, cuisine, and health. If you value what I have created here, I ask only one thing as a show of your appreciation. Please take a moment to visit the book's Amazon page (www.amazon.com/dp/B0741QQYT7), scroll past the product information to the customer reviews below, and click the "Write a customer review" button. Leave a short review (even a single sentence helps!) sharing your honest thoughts about what you have read. Having your review helps more than you could imagine with the process of getting more eyes on my work. Leaving a review is something anyone with an Amazon account can do, and it's incredibly effective for independent authors like myself. If you find value in a book, tell the world! Your voice matters.

Since publication, a number of readers have also reached out to me about interviews for their blogs, podcasts, and YouTube channels. I'm honored and humbled by these requests, and I've seen the big impact the publicity has had on spreading awareness of the book. I try to accommodate as many of these requests as possible, but I have had to rely on my daughter Anastasia to fill many of them in my stead, as she oversaw the majority of the translation from Ukrainian and production work. Please get in touch with her by email for any media inquiries such as these, and I am sure she will be happy to accommodate you. Reach her at: anastasia@identitypublications.com.

I hope the recipes in the *Extra Trim Edition* speak to you, cultivating intimacy and inspiring romance in your life. Food has been a vital part of the success of my marriage for the last three and a half decades, and I know many more couples stand to benefit from what it has done for me.

Olga Petrenko
July 2017
Kryvyi Rih, Ukraine

Original Preface

In this book, you will find fantastic recipes that will help you create and share intimate meals for and with your partner. It will help you understand which foods hold the power to help you create passionate meals and enhance lovemaking with someone you care for. I've gone out of my way to include scientific explanations about how and why these ingredients strongly affect human sexuality, as well as snippets which will enhance your appreciation of the recipes presented here.

By the time you've finished reading this book, you will have a new and informed understanding of what special roles ingredients, preparation, and planning play in the way you enjoy cooking.

Although it has taken me the better part of a decade to finish, I wrote *Intimacy On The Plate* with a very simple and clear purpose. It is to help lovers create a sensual and intimate meal without having to spend countless hours tracking down hard-to-find ingredients.

On these pages, you'll find everything you need in one convenient place:

- A clear explanation of what an aphrodisiac is.
- Which ingredients have aphrodisiac properties.
- How aphrodisiacs affect the sensuality of the mind and body.
- What you need to be aware of before using them in a dish.

- What specific effects they may have on yourself or the person you are cooking for.

The recipes presented in this book come from many diverse sources. Some are very rich and filling, while others are very light. I've included full-course meals as well as appetizers, snacks, and smaller entrées, so you will never run out of options for something to spice things up at home.

What each of the 200 recipes included here share is that they are all designed to awaken the sexually creative person within you. Used correctly, they will spur your imagination and enhance your hidden erotic nature. Your partner will enjoy both the artistry that goes into the flavor of each recipe, as well as the unique libido-enhancing qualities.

As with all meals, the effort put into the visual presentation is just as important as the preparation of the ingredients themselves – and especially so with the dishes I've included here. The visual aesthetic of a romantic meal has a strong influence on building sexual desire. Skillfully prepared ingredients and a beautifully served meal will raise both you and your partner's desires. It will prime you for an unforgettable sexual experience, highlighting the joy you are bound to experience together.

This book consists of six different sections, each focused on aphrodisiac foods which fall under particular major categories. Each category contains several chapters emphasizing specific ingredients which have their own unique erotic properties. This is done so that you may easily find the recipe you are looking for based on the foods you like and the ingredients you have available.

At the start of each section, you'll find brief descriptions for the erotic properties of each ingredient. Spend some time getting acquainted with the facts and figures behind each food before trying to create a magical meal with it.

These recipes are not set in stone. They exist only as a guide, and the motivation to pique your imagination. Figure out what you like about them, try new and exotic ideas, but do not forget about the traditional dishes proven by centuries of use around the world.

Introduction: What Are Aphrodisiacs?

The word "aphrodisiac" comes from the name of the Greek goddess of beauty and love, Aphrodite. Aphrodisiacs are any substances that increase libido when consumed. They do not address fertility issues or sexual dysfunction directly like certain little blue pills you may have heard of.

On the contrary, a meal created using aphrodisiac ingredients is a delicious feast created to contribute to awakening sexual desire and increasing attraction between two people. Combine the right timing and romantic atmosphere, and anyone can experience the power of aphrodisiacs in their own home any time they want.

Their legacy extends back through history. Emperors and kings used to eat oysters and raw eggs with ginseng root tincture before venturing to the marital bed.

The name of this book, *Intimacy On The Plate*, was chosen with great care. Nowadays, potent and romantic aphrodisiac dinners are available to each of us. Thanks to our modern understanding of the chemical composition of traditional ingredients, such as amino acids, vitamins, and trace elements, we now know exactly how they increase sexual activity naturally for both men and women.

While aphrodisiacs are the focus of this book, it is important that you do not forget about other erotic factors, such as lingerie, lighting, music, deep conversation, and the most important thing of all: attention to your partner. Japanese geisha believed that paying attention and displaying tenderness were the most powerful aphrodisiacs of all, and they should know.

I encourage you to go through this book with your loved one at your leisure and decide what to cook for your next romantic dinner. Open any chapter, and *voila* – you'll find recipes for every palate! You can cook them together, or prepare something on your own as a wonderful surprise for your partner. You'll also enjoy learning about the scientific theories contained here.

Male Aphrodisiacs

There is an ancient oriental proverb that states *"There is no better natural aphrodisiac for a man than a beautiful woman."* The proverb is wise, but in reality, things can be a bit more complex. Due to stress and age, an attractive beauty might not be enough to arouse a man's desires throughout his life. This is where aphrodisiacs come to the rescue, restoring the vitality to a man he may have been longing for since his youth.

There are three major types of aphrodisiacs for men: mineral, vegetable, and animal. For example, zinc is the most important trace element for the male body. It increases libido and male sex hormones. Seminal fluid can contain up to 2 milligrams per milliliter, and it can also be found in the prostate. Zinc plays a crucial role in the process of spermatogenesis and overall prostate function.

Zinc is a trace element which is required for sperm production. It also takes part in the metabolism of vitamin E, and is involved in the synthesis of various hormones, such as testosterone, insulin, and growth hormones. It also contributes to 500 different biochemical reactions in the human body.

Furthermore, zinc reduces the amount of aromatase enzyme in the male body. This molecule actually takes testosterone and turns it into the female sex hormone, estrogen. Zinc improves the efficiency of the signals sent by the pituitary gland to the testicles. This increases the amount of testosterone produced, as well as the effectiveness of the internal state of the testicles. This helps invigorate the sperm's endurance, effectively turning them into long distance swimmers. Just one or two oysters a day are enough to replenish the body's daily 15mg requirement of zinc in men.

Aphrodisiac medicines for men include Yohimbe, Impaza, Hippocampus Coronatus, and various other tonics.

Yohimbe is a medicine based on a substance extracted from the bark of the African Yohimbe tree. It improves blood flow to the genitals and increases sexual sensitivity. In addition, Yohimbe stimulates nerve centers of the brain that control sexuality. It leads to a sharp increase in receptor sensitivity, leaving fear and uncertainty behind. However, it doesn't have the same effect for people with low blood pressure. Yohimbe is purely a male aphrodisiac.

Impaza is a homeopathic medicine created from purified antibodies. It increases blood circulation to the genitals, which extends and enhances erections. If you take this medicine for a long time, the libido returns to normal and sexual satisfaction increases significantly.

Hippocampus Coronatus is a medicine consisting of seahorse extract, ginseng root extract, and kidney tea. It helps alleviate impotence, improves sexual stamina and libido, and intensifies orgasms.

Of all the aphrodisiac mediums, tonics affect men most slowly and gently - toning the entire body and contributing to the acceleration of the metabolic process. Tonics commonly contain extracts of ginseng root, Eleutherococcus, Aralia Manchu, and vitamins and trace elements.

A surprising food which is known to enhance potency is eggs, especially quail eggs. If you combine eggs with onions, they become an even greater aphrodisiac. In fact, adding garlic and onions to food was forbidden in monasteries because it could cause inappropriate sexual desire. Garlic contains a significant amount of selenium - a trace element responsible for male sexual health. In addition, it contains a stimulating substance called allicin.

The sexual temper of Italian men is well known all over the world. Italian food is rich in olive oil, garlic, roasted or steamed tomatoes, seafood, and various herbs, especially basil and celery. These foods stimulate and encourage passion and desire.

Nuts and seeds are also aphrodisiacs because they contain a high amount of vitamin E. In India, roasted sesame seeds are a traditional remedy for decreased potency when mixed with honey. People in Russia and the Ukraine mix walnuts with honey and take one dessert spoon 30 minutes after a meal to prepare them for a romantic encounter.

Siberian pine seeds, usually called pine nuts or pignoli, are a particularly strong aphrodisiac. The kernels of these nuts contain up to 66% fat and 20% protein. Due to the high protein content, pine nuts are also called love kernels. In addition to vitamins and trace elements, pine nuts also contain oleic acid, providing enough energy for any sexual encounter. Even the ancient Romans, recognized experts in comfort and pleasure, placed a high value on these and other seeds and nuts, and used them to improve their sexual health.

Celery is a powerful male aphrodisiac because it contains the male sex hormone androsterone, which enhances potency. Combined with sweat, it can have an arousing effect on women too. Parsley also has a positive effect on the balance of male hormones, as it contains apigenin which suppresses the female sex hormone, estrogen, in men.

Female Aphrodisiacs

In some ways, aphrodisiacs affect women quite differently than men. In other ways, they can be very similar.

You might be surprised to learn that one of the most popular aphrodisiacs for both women and men is an insect! It's known colloquially as Spanish Fly (Lytta vesicatoria), and it secretes a stimulating substance called cantharidin. Today Spanish Fly can be bought in pharmacies, clinics, and sex shops around the world as capsules, tinctures, powders, or drops. Cantharidin is odorless and tasteless and easily dissolved in beverages and food. In past centuries, people consumed the legs of frogs who had eaten Spanish Fly so that the effects would be passed along to them. One must be very careful when consuming Spanish Fly, however, as it has been known to act as a urinary tract irritant, even in low amounts, and some sources dispute its aphrodisiac powers.

Among herbal female aphrodisiacs, wormwood and ginseng stand out above the rest. They can be bought at pharmacies in the form of dried powders, tinctures, or capsules.

Ginkgo Biloba is rapidly gaining popularity among women too. This plant extract is commonly used to improve memory, but it also has sexually stimulating properties. Relaxing the blood vessel walls, it increases blood flow to the organs, especially the genitals. Thus, it increases sensitivity and, as a result, libido.

As with men, vanilla is a powerful sexual plant for women. Vanilla creates a feeling of comfort and peace, encouraging a sense of safety for a lot of women. If you are planning slow and exciting sex, you definitely should add a pinch of vanilla to your dessert or a drink.

Aloe Vera produces amino acids that stimulate blood flow to women's genitals. Juice from the leaves can be mixed with honey, and a single teaspoon daily of this mixture can be enough for most women. Aloe juice improves the rush of blood to the pelvic organs, enhancing sexual desire. The juice also contains antibodies and T-cells and is capable of restoring libido after surgery or injury.

Continue to Section I to learn more about how different kinds of vegetables and seasonings can enhance libido for both sexes.

Section I:
Vegetables, Mushrooms, Potherbs, & Seasonings

Vegetables are a vital component of any nutritious and healthy diet. Men looking to increase their sexual activity need a diverse diet based on a wide range of plants added to regular meals of meat and fish. Vegetables should generally be eaten raw in a 3:1 proportion with meat or fish. This is the most efficient ratio for revitalizing the male body and increasing potency. Vegetables, potherbs, and roots saturate the body with minerals, vitamins, essential oils, bio-stimulators, and bowel cleaners.

ARTICHOKES

This green king of love not only rejuvenates the body but also significantly increases sexual libido. The artichoke is unique too, as it is neither a fruit nor a vegetable, but a flower! In Arabic, it means earth thorn.

In ancient Rome and Greece artichokes were considered to be strong aphrodisiacs. People even credited them

cleanser of the body. It increases mental activity and normalizes hormonal balance. Celery contains the male hormone androsterone, which is responsible for erections.
When consumed, it changes the smell of male sweat, acting
as a pheromone which stimulates sexual desire in women.
Thanks to its diuretic properties, celery helps to cope with
infections of the genitourinary system and reproductive organs. All the parts of celery are extremely useful: the green
leaves, the stalk, and the root. However, the most useful
part is the root.

Celery is perfect for salads and it goes well with poultry,
fish, mushrooms, beans, eggplant, cabbage, and carrots.
Leafy celery or chive celery is used to decorate dishes. It
can be also added to soups, salads, or sauces. From celery
seeds you can create celery salt by mixing the seeds with
ordinary table salt.

SPINACH

Spinach originates from ancient Persia. The Arabs believed spinach was the king of vegetables. It was considered
a delicacy and only available to noble families. Spinach was
brought to Europe by the Crusaders during the Middle
Ages. The first harvest of this vegetable was collected by
Spanish monks who cultivated it in monastery gardens.

Nowadays, doctors recommend including spinach in the
diet of infertile women and impotent men. However, due
to the presence of oxalic acid, it cannot be consumed by
people suffering from rheumatism or gout.

Spinach is a vitamin champion. It contains 14 kinds of
vitamins and a large number of trace elements. These include B vitamins, biotin, vitamin C, tocopherol, calcium,

copper, and many others. Due to its composition, spinach improves one's mood, calms the nerves, stimulates synthesis of vital hormones, and stimulates the release of large amounts of androsterone.

ASPARAGUS

Once, asparagus was used to treat the prostate because it contains asparagine, which stimulates the functioning of the genitourinary tract. B vitamins, vitamin A, vitamin C, and the set of trace elements contained in asparagus enhance have a stimulating effect on sexual activity.

In France, there was a customary premarital practice of feeding the bride and groom three courses comprised of asparagus during the wedding dinner. Also, if you combine asparagus with wine you may avoid a hangover.

CABBAGE

All members of the cruciferous family of vegetables, including Brussels sprouts, cauliflower, kohlrabi, and red and green cabbages, are rich in vitamins and minerals. Even doctors of ancient Greece and Rome wrote about the healing properties of cabbage. They referred to it as a magical vegetable.

ROOT VEGETABLES

It is important to include beets, carrots, radishes, and turnips in your erotic menu. In fact, you should include turnips in your diet as often as possible because they activate bodily functions and increase potency. No wonder the humble turnip was considered the queen of the peasant table. To treat impotency, boil fresh turnip in carrot juice or

5

milk. Then grate it and mix with honey in a 1:1 ratio. Take one-third of a cup before each meal three times a day.

MUSHROOMS

Truffles and morels are considered to be the most potent mushrooms for increasing libido. Legend tells us that morels were respected by Casanova, while Angelique, the main temptress of Anne and Serge Golon's novels, preferred truffles. A legendary nymphomaniac, Messalina, used to feed her lovers the same mushroom delicacy. In addition to morels and truffles, wild mushrooms also have aphrodisiac properties, but only the ones grown in a natural environment.

Mushrooms have always been a mysterious and even shamanistic food. They have a lot of protein and zinc, which are well-known components needed to increase sexual energy. Zinc is involved in sperm production and testosterone synthesis. Truffles are exceptional because they contain a combination of macro element phosphoresces. This is a component of lecithin which is involved in the formation of gametes.

ALLIUMS

Alliums include onions, chives, leek, spring onion, rock onion, shallot, and garlic. Given the smell of onions, you might not think they would be aphrodisiacs. The offending smell and taste of onions and garlic in the mouth can be neutralized by parsley or mint. Just chew on a sprig to remove the noxious odor. The majority of men intuitively like onions and garlic. Both foods contain a lot of zinc and selenium, which restore the body's hormonal balance. Garlic contains large amounts of allicin, which is a substance that stimulates certain parts of the brain.

PARSLEY

Parsley is very useful for men who are experiencing impotency, as it contains a substance called apigenin. This inhibits the production of the female sex hormone estrogen in men. In addition, apigenin is an antioxidant. Parsley normalizes the adrenal glands, which also produce the male hormone testosterone. Parsley contains vitamins A, B3, C, and K, as well as essential oils and the minerals potassium, calcium, zinc, iron, and magnesium. This classic herb is suitable for almost all dishes, except sweet ones, and makes a wonderful garnish for nearly any meal.

POTHERBS

Potherbs include purslane, basil, tarragon, savory, thyme, St. John's wort, anise, caraway, tarragon, marjoram, parsley, and dill. From early spring to late autumn, you can include the leaves of raspberry, currant, strawberry, rose, oak, and linden in your romantic dinner menu. They all contain a high amount of nutrients and bowel cleansers. Additionally, their forest fragrance can excite the surliest of men and raise his spirits. Simply wash them, dry them on a paper towel, and finely chop the leaves. Then add them to a dish just like you would any other potherb.

001 Roman Artichokes

INGREDIENTS

4 MAMMOLE ARTICHOKES
1 CLOVE OF GARLIC
1 BUNCH OF PARSLEY
A FEW LEAVES OF LEMON BALM
2 TBSP OF BREADCRUMBS
1 TBSP OF OLIVE OIL
JUICE OF ½ LEMON
SALT & PEPPER
3.5 OZ (100G) OF ANCHOVIES FOR SERVING

PREPARATION

Remove the leaves from each artichoke, leaving only the core with 5cm of stem. Clean the core of all fibers ("hairs"). Grind the garlic, parsley, and lemon balm, and mix them with the breadcrumbs and olive oil. Stuff the artichokes with breadcrumb mixture. Place the prepared artichokes into a deep pan upside down. Pour water and olive oil in a 1:1 ratio over the artichokes. Simmer everything under a closed lid for 10 minutes over medium heat, followed by 20 minutes over low heat.

SERVING

Place 2 artichokes on each plate. Serve anchovies as a side dish.

002 Tortilla with Artichokes

INGREDIENTS

4 BOILED ARTICHOKES
VEGETABLE OIL FOR FRYING
4 EGGS
SALT & PEPPER
POTHERBS FOR SERVING

PREPARATION

Cut boiled artichokes into pieces. Fry them in vegetable oil until golden brown. Beat the eggs with a fork until smooth, and add salt to taste.

Take two prepared artichokes for one portion, and pour them over with half the egg mixture. Spread evenly over the pan and cover it with a lid. After 2 minutes, flip it to the other side. Continue frying for 2 more minutes. Then cook the second serving.

SERVING

Place a tortilla on each serving plate. Decorate the dish with your favorite potherbs.

003 Shades of Flavor Salad

INGREDIENTS

21 OZ (600G) OF ARTICHOKES
SALT & GROUND PEPPER
3.5 OZ (100G) OF PARMESAN CHEESE
1 APPLE
1 LEMON
4 TBSP OF OLIVE OIL
1 BUNCH OF SPRING ONIONS

PREPARATION

Remove the inedible parts of the artichoke, and cut it into small pieces. Boil for 15 minutes. Cut the parmesan cheese into very thin slices with a vegetable peeler. Slice the apples and sprinkle them with lemon juice. To prepare a sauce, mix lemon juice, olive oil, and black pepper. Combine the artichokes with the apples and dress them as you desire with the sauce.

SERVING

Lay out the apples and artichokes on a serving plate and cover them with cheese slices. Sprinkle the dish with chopped green onions.

004 Avocado Stuffed Artichokes

INGREDIENTS

4 ARTICHOKES
JUICE OF ½ LEMON
9 OZ (250G) 33% FAT CREAM
1 AVOCADO
3.5 OZ (100G) SALAMI
2 OZ (50G) PARMESAN CHEESE
A PINCH OF OREGANO
SALT
BOILED RICE FOR A SIDE DISH

PREPARATION

Clean the artichokes by removing the leaves and fibers, and put them in boiling salted water. Add lemon juice and lemon zest. Let boil for 20 minutes. Remove from heat, drain the water, and let it cool. To prepare the stuffing, whip the cream and mix with avocado, finely chopped salami, grated cheese, lemon juice, oregano, and salt. Fill the artichoke cores with stuffing.

SERVING

Put two artichokes on each serving plate. Place a serving of boiled rice beside the artichokes. Sprinkle the whole dish with oregano.

005 Heady Artichokes

INGREDIENTS

4 ARTICHOKES
OLIVE OIL FOR FRYING
1 CUP DRY WHITE WINE
YOUR FAVORITE POTHERBS
SALT & PEPPER

PREPARATION

First, clean the artichokes. You will need to smooth them out, removing all hairs and inedible parts. Cut the prepared artichokes into two pieces and fry them in olive oil. Pour dry wine over them and season with spices, salt, and pepper. Keep simmering until the wine has evaporated.

SERVING

Lay the artichokes out on a large platter. Serve with white wine.

Tip: Artichokes and asparagus are vegetables, and are not always easy to choose wine for. The Spanish wine Mas de les Valls goes best with artichoke dishes. Californian white wines also work well.

006 Piquant Pumpkin

INGREDIENTS

14 OZ (400G) OF PUMPKIN PULP
2 TBSP OF APPLE CIDER VINEGAR
1 TSP OF HONEY
1 SPRIG OF ROSEMARY
1 TSP OF DIJON MUSTARD
2 TBSP OF OLIVE OIL
SALT & GROUND BLACK PEPPER
1 TBSP OF SESAME SEEDS
2 OZ (50G) OF BLUE CHEESE
DILL & PARSLEY FOR SERVING

PREPARATION

Cut the pumpkin into bars. Prepare the marinade by mixing 1 teaspoon of vinegar with the honey, rosemary, mustard, and olive oil. Season the pumpkin bars with salt and pepper, then pour the marinade over it. Set aside for 1 hour. Put the pumpkin and marinade into a heated pan. Once the marinade has evaporated, add the sesame seeds and keep frying for 1 more minute. When done, sprinkle with the remaining vinegar.

SERVING

Place pumpkin on 2 serving plates. Sprinkle with crumbled cheese and potherbs.

007 Magic Pumpkin

INGREDIENTS

17.5 OZ (500G) OF ORANGE PUMPKIN PULP
1 TSP OF ITALIAN POTHERBS
1 OZ (30G) OF OLIVE OIL
1 TBSP OF PUMPKIN SEEDS
2 OZ (50G) OF BLUE CHEESE
A FEW LEAVES OF ARUGULA
A HANDFUL OF WALNUTS
FRESHLY GROUND PEPPER

PREPARATION

Cut the pumpkin pulp with a cheese knife into small squares approx. 1" (2.5cm) long. Sprinkle them with dried Italian potherbs. Preheat the oven to 350°F (180°C). Put the pumpkin on a baking sheet and bake until tender for approx. 15 minutes. Slightly fry the pumpkin seeds or dry them in the oven.

SERVING

Place the pumpkin bars on a platter. Sprinkle with crumbled cheese, and decorate with arugula and pumpkin seeds. Season the dish with pepper using a mill.

14

008 Pumpkin with Smoked Bacon & Cherry Sauce

INGREDIENTS

8 SLICES OF TURKEY BREAST OF THE SAME SIZE
SALT & PEPPER
8 PUMPKIN BARS APPROX. 3" X 1" (8CM X 3CM)
8 SMALL SPRIGS OF SAVORY & ROSEMARY
8 SLICES OF SMOKED BACON
2 OR 3 TYPES OF NUTS FOR SERVING

SAUCE:
3.5 OZ (100G) OF PITTED CHERRIES
1 TBSP OF RED WINE
½ TSP OF CARDAMOM

PREPARATION

Season the turkey pieces with salt and pepper, and then fry them in a grilled pan from both sides. Put a piece of turkey on each pumpkin bar. Lay out a sprig of savory on top of it and cover everything with bacon. Bake at 350°F (180°C) for 20 minutes.

To prepare the sauce: blend the cherries and then add the wine and cardamom. Bring everything to a boil in a saucepan and then remove from heat.

SERVING

Take 2 big plates and place 4 pumpkin rolls on each. Form tracks of the sauce on one side of each plate in front of each roll. Spread the nuts on the other side.

009 Pumpkin Carpaccio

INGREDIENTS

7 OZ (200G) OF PUMPKIN PULP
1 OZ (30G) OF PARMESAN CHEESE
A FEW SPRIGS OF ARUGULA
2 OZ (50G) OF SESAME OIL
A PINCH OF BLACK PEPPER MIGNONETTE

PREPARATION

Cut the pumpkin into thin strips. Bake them in the oven at 350°F (180°C) for 5 minutes.

SERVING

Serve the dish on a large platter. Lay out the pumpkin petals around the platter, filling out the entire plate. Place grated cheese on the rim of the plate, and put arugula in the center of the dish. Sprinkle the carpaccio with sesame oil and season with black pepper mignonette.

010 Pumpkin Under Chocolate Chips

INGREDIENTS

17.5 OZ (500G) OF PUMPKIN PULP
2 OZ (60G) OF BUTTER
4 OZ (120G) OF PITTED PRUNES
3 TBSP OF SUGAR
A HANDFUL OF DRIED CHERRIES OR CRANBERRIES
FOR SERVING
1 OZ (30G) OF DARK CHOCOLATE CHIPS
1 OZ (30G) OF WHITE CHOCOLATE CHIPS

PREPARATION

Cut the pumpkin pulp into small cubes. Grease the bottom of a baking dish with butter. Put the pumpkin in it and place prunes on top of it, follow by another layer of pumpkin. Cover the top with sugar and fill ⅓ of the dish with water. Cover the dish with a lid or foil. Bake at 350°F (180°C) for 40 minutes.

SERVING

Equally spread the pumpkin and prunes into 2 rectangular salad bowls. Decorate with dried berries. Sprinkle with black and white chocolate chips.

011 Sweet Root Salad

INGREDIENTS

2 OZ (50G) OF CELERY ROOT
1 SOUR GREEN APPLE
1 TBSP OF YOGURT
½ TSP OF DIJON MUSTARD
½ TSP OF HONEY
SALT
1 SPRIG OF POTHERBS FOR SERVING

PREPARATION

Cut the raw celery root into strips or grate it. Slice the apple into strips. To prepare the dressing, mix the yogurt with mustard, honey, and salt. Combine the celery, apple, and dressing.

SERVING

Lay out the salad using a culinary ring. Decorate with a sprig of any potherb.

012 Vitamin Hill Salad

INGREDIENTS

7 OZ (200G) OF CELERY STALK
7 OZ (200G) OF COOKED PUMPKIN
2 APPLES
½ LEMON
2 OZ (50G) OF WALNUTS
2 TBSP OF OLIVE OIL
4 TBSP OF HONEY
3 TBSP OF PARTRIDGE BERRIES OR CRANBERRIES
A HANDFUL OF CRANBERRIES
A SPRIG OF PARSLEY OR A CELERY LEAF
1 LEMON SLICE FOR SERVING

PREPARATION

Cut the celery, pumpkin, and apples into strips. Sprinkle the apples with lemon juice.

To prepare the dressing, mix walnuts (lightly roasted), olive oil, honey, and partridge berries or cranberries in a blender. Dress the salad with this mixture.

SERVING

Place the salad onto a large round or oval dish. Sprinkle with a handful of berries. Place a sprig of green potherbs on top of the salad and a slice of lemon beside it.

013 Spicy Celery Salad

INGREDIENTS

3.5 OZ (100G) OF PEELED CELERY ROOT
1 LEEK
1 BUNCH OF SPRING ONIONS
A BUNCH OF PARSLEY OR DILL
1 APPLE
1 LEMON
1 CAN OF TUNA
1 TBSP OF MAYONNAISE
6 WALNUT HALVES
A SPRIG OF ANY POTHERBS FOR SERVING

PREPARATION

Cut or grate the celery. Chop the leek, spring onion, and parsley or dill very finely. Cut the apple into small cubes and sprinkle it with lemon juice. Combine the apples with the mixed vegetables and potherbs. Add canned tuna and a spoonful of mayonnaise, and then mix everything thoroughly.

SERVING

Put the salad into dessert bowls. Lay out the walnuts halves and a sprig of green potherbs on top of the salad.

014 Celery & Chicken Soufflé

INGREDIENTS

5.5 OZ (150G) OF CELERY ROOT
14 OZ (400G) OF CHICKEN FILLETS
1 ONION
2 TBSP OF BUTTER
2 TBSP OF RICE FLOUR
A PINCH OF NUTMEG
SALT & FRESHLY GROUND PEPPER
2 EGGS
3.5 TBSP OF 20% FAT CREAM
2 SPRIGS OF CELERY GREENS FOR SERVING

PREPARATION

Boil peeled celery root until tender (approx. 20 minutes). Remove the celery from heat and puree it. Mince the chicken fillets or blend them in a blender. Finely chop the onions and fry them in butter. Combine mashed celery, onion, chicken, and rice flour. Season the mix with salt, nutmeg, and pepper. Beat the eggs with cream and add them to the prepared chicken mix. Grease the soufflé molds with butter. Lay out the mix into the molds. Place them into a deep baking pan with a little water. Bake at 350°F (180°C) for 40 minutes.

SERVING

Place hot soufflé on coasters. Decorate with celery leaf.

015 Coleslaw with Celery & Apple

INGREDIENTS

1 CUP OF WALNUTS
28 OZ (800G) OF CELERY ROOT
2.5 TBSP OF APPLE VINEGAR
14 OZ (400G) OF RED APPLES
½ CUP OF DRIED CRANBERRIES
7 FL OZ (200 ML) OF 10% FAT SOUR CREAM
2 TSP OF HORSERADISH
1.5 TSP OF DIJON MUSTARD
1 TSP OF SUGAR
SALT & PEPPER
CELERY FOR SERVING

PREPARATION

Dry the nuts in the oven and coarsely chop them. Peel the celery root and cut it into strips. Pour 2 tbsp of apple vinegar over it, and thoroughly mix everything. Remove the core from the apples and cut them into thin slices. Combine the celery, apples, walnuts, and cranberries. Whip sour cream, horseradish, mustard, 1.5 teaspoons of vinegar, salt, and pepper in a separate bowl. Season the salad with this sauce and refrigerate for a couple of hours.

SERVING

Lay out the salad into square salad bowls. Decorate the dish with celery greens.

016 Spinach Balls a la Tempera

INGREDIENTS

14 OZ (400G) OF SPINACH
VEGETABLE OIL & BUTTER FOR FRYING
3 CLOVES OF GARLIC
9 OZ (250G) OF COD FILLET
4 TBSP OF FLOUR
13.5 FL OZ (400 ML) OF MILK
1 CUP OF BREADCRUMBS
1 LARGE EGG
CRANBERRIES & LETTUCE LEAVES FOR SERVING

PREPARATION

Fry spinach in butter for 6 minutes. Mix in a blender. Roast garlic cloves whole. Remove garlic from pan and fry minced cod fillets for 2 minutes in garlic oil. Add spinach and gradually pour flour diluted in milk. Let simmer and stir constantly with a wooden spoon until thick. Move the mixture to a bowl and allow it to cool slightly. Form balls from spinach-cod mixture with a dessert spoon. Roll the balls in breadcrumbs, then beaten egg, before rolling in breadcrumbs once more. Fry the balls in vegetable oil for 3-4 minutes. Put them on a paper towel.

SERVING

Lay out the lettuce leaves on a serving plate. Put the spinach balls in a row on top of the lettuce. To decorate the dish, randomly spread the cranberries around the plate.

017 Pkhali Spinach

INGREDIENTS

7 OZ (200G) OF FRESH SPINACH
BUTTER FOR FRYING
½ CUP OF WALNUTS
SPICES (CILANTRO, CORIANDER, & DILL)
2 CLOVES OF GARLIC
WINE VINEGAR TO TASTE
1 TOMATO
2 BOILED QUAIL EGGS
POMEGRANATE SEEDS

PREPARATION

Boil the spinach for one minute or fry it in butter. Then blend it in a blender. Grind nuts with spices in a blender as well. Combine all the ingredients and season them with wine vinegar.

SERVING

Form the prepared mixture into small balls. Put 3 balls on a serving dish. Lay out finely chopped crosswise tomatoes on one side of the plate, and quail eggs on the other. To decorate the dish, sprinkle the spinach balls with pomegranate seeds.

018 Italian Baked Spinach Sea Bass

INGREDIENTS

4 FL OZ (120 ML) OF DRY WHITE WINE
1 BAY LEAF
2 SEA BASS FILLETS
2 ONIONS
1.5 FL OZ (40 ML) OF VEGETABLE OIL
25 OZ (700G) OF SPINACH
A PINCH OF NUTMEG
SALT & GROUND WHITE PEPPER
1 LEMON
A HANDFUL OF SESAME SEEDS FOR SERVING

PREPARATION

Pour the wine into a saucepan. Add the bay leaf and bring everything to a boil. Put fish fillets into the saucepan and cook for 10 minutes. Move the sea bass into a bowl. Chop the onions and fry them in butter. Add the spinach, nutmeg, salt, and pepper. Simmer everything for 8 minutes. Lay out the fillets into a baking dish, and place the spinach and lemon slices on top of the fish. Pour the broth over it. Bake the fish in an oven at 425°F (220°C) for 10 minutes.

SERVING

Lay out the sea bass with spinach on 2 rectangular dishes. Sprinkle the dish with roasted sesame seeds.

019 Spinach Shrimp with Japanese Motifs

INGREDIENTS

2 TOMATOES
14 OZ (400G) OF SPINACH
21 OZ (600G) OF SHRIMP
2 CLOVES OF GARLIC
1 TBSP OF CHOPPED PARSLEY
½ TSP OF LEMON ZEST
1 TBSP OF LEMON JUICE
½ TSP OF BLACK PEPPER
2 TBSP OF OLIVE OIL
PARSLEY FOR SERVING
2 UNPEELED SHRIMP

PREPARATION

Chop the tomatoes and spinach. Add vegetable oil and salt. Take 2 baking dishes and evenly spread the vegetables. Peel the shrimp and season them with salt, garlic, parsley, lemon zest, lemon juice, and pepper. Pour the olive oil. Put the shrimp on a tomato-spinach bed. Bake in the oven at 350°F (180°C) for 20 minutes. Fry 2 shrimp with their shells in vegetable oil.

SERVING

Serve the dish in the same molds they were baked in. Decorate with chopped potherbs and place unpeeled fried shrimp on top of each mold.

020 Pyramid Salad

INGREDIENTS

1 ROASTED BEET
1 RAW CARROT
1 TOMATO
5.5 OZ (150G) OF FRESH SPINACH
5.5 OZ (150G) OF ARUGULA
1 TSP OF SESAME SEEDS
A HANDFUL OF SPROUTED WHEAT GRAINS

DRESSING:
1 TSP OF OLIVE OIL
DILL
BASIL
SALT
1 TBSP OF APPLE CIDER VINEGAR

PREPARATION

Wash beet and wrap it in foil. Bake it in the oven at 350°F (180°C) for 1 hour. Cut the cooked beet into strips. Grate the carrot and slice the tomato into cubes. Mix all the ingredients in a bowl. Add the spinach. To season the salad, prepare the sauce by mixing olive oil, spices, salt, and vinegar.

SERVING

Lay out the salad in the form of a pyramid on a serving dish. Randomly place the arugula leaves on top of the pyramid and sprinkle it with lightly fried sesame seeds.

021 Italian Asparagus Salad with Grapefruit

INGREDIENTS

14 OZ (400G) OF ASPARAGUS
14 OZ (400G) OF GRAPEFRUIT
7 OZ (200G) OF PREPARED & PEELED SHRIMP
1 TBSP OF OLIVE OIL
JUICE OF ½ LEMON
SALT & PEPPER
4 LETTUCE LEAVES
1 TSP OF CHOPPED PARSLEY FOR SERVING

PREPARATION

Tie the asparagus up into a bunch and boil for 5 minutes. Cut it into slices. Divide the grapefruit into slices and remove any bitter white film. Mix the asparagus, grapefruit slices, and shrimp. Season the salad with olive oil, salt, and pepper.

SERVING

Lay out 2 lettuce leaves on each serving plate. Place the salad on top of the lettuce and sprinkle it with potherbs.

022 Masa-Barmas Salad

INGREDIENTS

1 ZUCCHINI
4 ASPARAGUS STALKS
4 CHERRY TOMATOES
1 TBSP OF OLIVE OIL
4 SCALLOPS
1 TSP OF LEMON JUICE
1 TBSP OF JAPANESE SPICES
1 TSP OF GREEN PEAS OR WHEAT SPROUTS
SALT & PEPPER

PREPARATION

Peel the zucchini with a vegetable peeler or zest grater. Remove the seeds and cut into slices ½ inch thick. Remove the tough rinds from the asparagus stalks and slice them diagonally. Cut the cherry tomatoes into rings. Boil the asparagus for 4 minutes and the zucchini slices for 2 minutes. Move the vegetables into the ice water with a slotted spoon, so that the vegetables keep their color. Dry them on a paper towel. Heat the oil in a frying pan and fry the scallops for 1 minute on each side. Turn off the heat, close the lid, and leave it for 10 minutes. Slightly warm the asparagus and zucchini before serving.

SERVING

Spread out the vegetables on two serving plates. Place two scallops on each plate. Sprinkle the dish with lemon juice and generously season it with Japanese spices.

023 Warm White Asparagus Salad

INGREDIENTS

21 OZ (600G) OF WHITE ASPARAGUS
1 ORANGE
10.5 OZ (300G) OF ARUGULA
½ CUP OF DRIED WALNUTS
1 TBSP OF LEMON JUICE
3 TBSP OF OLIVE OIL
1 TSP OF PINE NUTS
A PINCH OF SAFFRON

PREPARATION

Steam the asparagus for 5 minutes, and then peel and cut it into 2" pieces. Divide the orange into slices and remove any bitter film. Mix the asparagus, orange slices, arugula, and walnuts. Season the salad with lemon juice and olive oil.

SERVING

Place the salad on two large flat plates. Sprinkle the dish with pine nuts and saffron.

024 Striking Night Salad

INGREDIENTS

2 SMALL SQUIDS
5.5 OZ (150G) OF ASPARAGUS
1 MANGO
1 AVOCADO
PINE NUTS FOR SERVING
FLAKES OF RED PEPPER

DRESSING:
1 FL OZ (30 ML) OF OLIVE OIL
1 TSP OF DIJON MUSTARD
2 TBSP OF LEMON JUICE
1 TSP OF WHITE VINEGAR
½ TSP OF SESAME OIL
1 TSP OF SOY SAUCE
A PINCH OF DRIED RED PEPPER
1 TSP OF ROASTED PINE NUTS
A PINCH OF SUGAR

PREPARATION

Boil the squids for 2 minutes. Let them cool and cut them into thin rings. Cut the asparagus into squares and boil in salted water. Peel the mango and avocado and cut them into cubes. Mix the asparagus with squid, avocado, and mango.

To prepare the dressing: mix all the ingredients and pour it over the salad. Refrigerate the salad for 30 minutes.

SERVING

Lay out the asparagus salad on 2 flat plates. Sprinkle the dish with pine nuts and pepper flakes.

025 Asparagus Rolls

INGREDIENTS

1 ZUCCHINI
4 STALKS OF GREEN ASPARAGUS
3.5 OZ (100G) OF GREEN BEANS
8 GREEN PEA PODS
4 SMALL SALMON FILLETS
2 TBSP OF OLIVE OIL
SALT

SPICY SAUCE:
PARSLEY
A SMALL BUNCH OF CILANTRO
TARRAGON
¼ TSP OF CORIANDER SEEDS
SALT
3.5 FL OZ (100 ML) OF OLIVE OIL
1 FL OZ (30 ML) OF BALSAMIC VINEGAR

PREPARATION

Peel the zucchini and cut it into thin slices. Separately boil all the vegetables and place them into ice water to preserve color.

To prepare the spicy sauce: tie the potherbs into a bunch. Boil them in a small amount of water with coriander seeds and a pinch of sea salt. Strain the broth, and then add olive oil and vinegar. Place it into the fridge.

To make the rolls, cover the zucchini slices with plastic wrap. Place asparagus slices and pea pods in the middle of the dish and wrap it up. Tightly fix the edges of the plastic wrap and refrigerate the rolls for 30 minutes.

Fry the salmon fillets on both sides in olive oil.

SERVING

Place the vegetable rolls on 2 large plates. Cover the bottom of the dish with the spicy sauce. Then, lay out the fish and pour the sauce over it.

026 Podium Salad

INGREDIENTS

3 OZ (90G) OF BUTTER
2 OZ (50G) OF ROASTED HAZELNUTS
1 ORANGE
2LBS (1KG) OF BRUSSELS SPROUTS
12.5 OZ (350G) OF FROZEN PEAS

PREPARATION

Soften the butter at room temperature. Add hazelnut and the zest from the orange. Cut the Brussels sprouts in ½ and boil in salted water for 5 minutes. Boil the peas separately from the Brussels sprouts. Mix the peas and Brussels sprouts, and season the salad with orange oil.

SERVING

Lay out the Brussels sprouts and peas on a dish using a culinary ring. Pour orange juice in zigzag movements over the dish.

027 Kohlrabi Salad

INGREDIENTS

1 KOHLRABI OF ANY TYPE
1" (2CM) OF FRESH GRATED GINGER ROOT
3 TBSP OF OLIVE OIL
3 TBSP OF BALSAMIC VINEGAR
SALT
2 TSP OF LIQUID HONEY
½ TSP OF DRIED ITALIAN POTHERBS
4 TBSP OF DRIED SESAME SEEDS & PARSLEY FOR
SERVING

PREPARATION

Grate the kohlrabi Korean style and add ginger root to it.
To prepare the sauce: mix olive oil with balsamic vinegar,
salt, honey, spicy dried potherbs, and salt. Season the salad
with this dressing. Leave it for 30 minutes.

SERVING

Lay out the salad into a square bowl. To decorate the dish,
sprinkle the salad with sesame seeds and parsley.

028 Radicchio & Cauliflower Salad

INGREDIENTS

10.5 OZ (300G) OF RADICCHIO OR ITALIAN CHIC-ORY
2 SHALLOTS
2 TBSP OF RAISINS
1 OZ (30G) OF ANCHOVIES
1 CAULIFLOWER
2 TBSP OF PINE NUTS
¼ TBSP OF OLIVE OIL
2 TBSP OF WHITE WINE VINEGAR
A HANDFUL OF DRIED PINE NUTS FOR SERVING

PREPARATION

Peel the radicchio and cut it into thin strips. Finely chop the onion. Soak the raisins in hot water for 10 minutes. Drain the water and dry the raisins. Wash and clean the anchovies. Separate the cauliflower into florets and boil them until they are cooked. Fry the onions, raisins, and nuts in the olive oil in a saucepan for 8 minutes. Add the anchovies and let cook another 3 minutes. Add the vinegar and 1 tbsp of water. Simmer all the ingredients for one more minute. Mix the cauliflower and radicchio with the contents of the saucepan.

SERVING

The salad is served in a deep platter, sprinkled with roasted pine nuts.

029 Gourmet Cauliflower

INGREDIENTS

10 FL OZ (300 ML) OF GREEK YOGHURT
JUICE OF 1 LIME
2 TBSP OF CHILI POWDER
1 TBSP OF CRUSHED GARLIC
1 TBSP OF CUMIN
1 TSP OF SALT
½ TSP OF BLACK PEPPER
1 TSP OF CURRY POWDER
1 CAULIFLOWER
1 TBSP OF VEGETABLE OIL
LETTUCE LEAVES FOR SERVING

PREPARATION

Mix the yogurt, lime juice, chili powder, garlic, cumin, salt, pepper, and curry powder. Thoroughly cover the cauliflower with this mixture. Preheat the oven to 400°F (200°C). Grease the baking dish with vegetable oil and place the whole cauliflower on it. Bake for 40 minutes. The marinade will give a delicious crust to the cauliflower.

SERVING

Cover a large platter with lettuce leaves. Slice the cauliflower just like a cake.

030 Sherry Sauerkraut

INGREDIENTS

1 RED CABBAGE
1.5 FL OZ (45 ML) OF RED WINE VINEGAR
2.5 FL OZ (75 ML) OF SHERRY
3.5 OZ (100G) OF SMOKED BACON
SALT & PEPPER
1 TBSP OF SUGAR
1 APPLE
½ TSP OF THYME
4 FRIED SAUSAGES FOR THE SIDE DISH

PREPARATION

Chop the red cabbage into sticks and pour the vinegar marinade and a tbsp of sherry over it. Mash the cabbage with your hands for 7-8 minutes. Leave it to marinate in the fridge for 24 hours. Cut the bacon into strips and fry until golden brown. Add red cabbage and simmer for 15 minutes. Add some salt, sugar, pepper, vinegar, and sherry. Let simmer for 15 more minutes. Cut the apple into cubes. Add it and thyme to the dish.

SERVING

Place the sauerkraut on 2 individual dishes. Use 2 sausages per serving as a side dish.

031 Erotic Baked Mushrooms

INGREDIENTS

10 FRESH MUSHROOMS
1 CARROT
1 TBSP OF CHOPPED TURNIP
1 CUP OF CHOPPED CABBAGE
SALT
2 FL OZ (60 ML) OF SOUR CREAM
PARSLEY FOR SERVING

PREPARATION

Clean and chop the mushrooms. Cut the carrot and turnip into thin strips. Mix the vegetables with the mushrooms, salt, and sour cream. Add the mixture to boiling water and cook over medium heat for 7 minutes. Remove from heat and let flavors continue to infuse for 12 minutes.

SERVING

Lay everything out on a dish. Pour a little broth over it, and sprinkle with finely chopped parsley.

032 Belgian Salad with Tartar Sauce

INGREDIENTS

9 OZ (250G) OF FRESH MUSHROOMS
3 TBSP OF OLIVE OIL
1 CELERY STALK
9 OZ (250G) OF COOKED & FROZEN MUSSELS
SALT & PEPPER
PARSLEY FOR SERVING

TARTAR SAUCE:
1 TSP OF PICKLED CUCUMBERS
1 TSP OF SPRING ONIONS
2 TBSP OF MAYONNAISE
1 TSP OF CAPERS
½ TSP OF LEMON JUICE
¼ TSP OF DIJON MUSTARD
¼ TSP OF WORCESTERSHIRE SAUCE
¼ TSP OF DRIED TARRAGON
½ TSP OF CHOPPED PARSLEY

PREPARATION

Slice mushrooms. Fry in olive oil. Cut celery root and boil. Thaw mussels. Rinse and dry. Mix all ingredients.

To prepare the tartar sauce: finely chop pickled cucumbers and spring onions. Mix with remaining ingredients.

SERVING

Put the salad into 2 serving dishes. Sprinkle with parsley.

41

033 Cold Mushroom Tangerine Mood Appetizer

INGREDIENTS

3.5 OZ (100G) OF MUSHROOMS
2 APPLES
6 TANGERINES
2 SWEET PEPPERS
7 OZ (200G) OF CHEESE

SAUCE:
7 FL OZ (200 ML) OF GREEK YOGHURT
1 TSP OF MUSTARD
1 TSP OF LIQUID HONEY
JUICE OF ½ LEMON

PREPARATION

Slice the mushrooms and boil them until tender for 15 minutes. Peel the apples and cut them into cubes. Remove the white film from 5 tangerines and then divide them into segments. Cut the peppers into rings. Mix all ingredients.

To prepare the sauce: mix yogurt, mustard, honey, and lemon juice in a blender. Season the salad with the sauce.

SERVING

Place the salad in a beautiful salad bowl. Use tangerine slices to make a ring around the bowl.

034 The Highway Dish

INGREDIENTS

17.5 OZ (500G) OF FRESH MUSHROOMS
1 ONION
3.5 OZ (100G) OF PEELED PEANUTS
2 FL OZ (50 ML) OF VEGETABLE OR PEANUT OIL
SALT
MUSHROOM SPICES
2 TBSP OF POMEGRANATE SEEDS FOR SERVING

SIDE DISH:
1 HEAD OF BROCCOLI
1 RED GRAPEFRUIT
SALT & PEPPER TO TASTE

SAUCE:
1 RED ONION
½ CUP OF DRIED WALNUTS HALVES
1 TBSP OF HONEY
1 TBSP OF OLIVE OIL
2 TBSP OF WHITE WINE VINEGAR

PREPARATION

Wash the mushrooms and cut them into four quarters. Slice the onion into small cubes. Crush 2 oz (50g) of peanuts with a rolling pin. Heat the oil. Lightly fry the onion, and then add whole and crushed peanuts into the frying pan. Continue frying the onion and peanuts for a couple of minutes. Add mushrooms. Season with salt and mushroom spices. Simmer for 15 minutes to evaporate the liquid.

To prepare the side dish: divide the broccoli into florets. Fry them for approx. 1 minute, and then move them into a bowl with ice water to preserve the color. Remove any white film from the grapefruit and separate it into segments. To make a dressing for the salad, mix finely chopped onion and walnuts with honey, olive oil, and wine vinegar. Mix the broccoli florets and grapefruit, and then season the salad with this dressing. Add salt and pepper to your taste.

SERVING

Lay out mushrooms and bright salad strips opposite each other on a serving plate. Sprinkle the salad with pomegranate seeds.

035 Stir Fried Mushrooms

INGREDIENTS

17.5 OZ (500G) OF CHICKEN FILLETS
½ TBSP OF OYSTER SAUCE
1 TBSP OF CORNSTARCH
2 TBSP OF PEANUT BUTTER
A FEW SPRING ONIONS
8 SLICES OF PEELED GINGER
2 CLOVES OF GARLIC
10 OZ (300G) OF ANY MUSHROOM
10 OZ (300G) OF BOK CHOY SALAD
10 FL OZ (300 ML) OF BROTH
2 TSP OF SESAME OIL
4 PIECES OF TOAST FOR SERVING

PREPARATION

Marinate chicken pieces in oyster sauce. Dilute the starch in 3 tablespoons of cold water. Heat the wok or any other deep frying pan over high heat and add peanut oil. Add chopped spring onions, ginger, and finely chopped garlic. Fry this mix for 12-15 seconds. Add the chicken to the pan and continue frying for 3 more minutes. When finished, add the mushrooms and bok choy salad. Pour broth over it. Add sesame oil and bring everything to a boil. Add the starch, and stir-fry the dish for 3 minutes until thickened.

SERVING

Serve the dish with toast in deep bowls.

Section II: Fish

Although many types of shellfish and other seafood are well known as aphrodisiacs, the same association is not usually shared by regular fish. You probably know that fish can be excellent sources of vitamins, proteins, fats, minerals and trace elements which benefit the entire body. Did you also know they contain phosphorus, which promotes the formation of healthy sperm and enhances sexual desire? Saltwater fish, in particular, contain the highest amount of phosphorus. Additionally, protein gives the body strength and endurance, while iodine improves one's mood and sexual desire by assisting the function of the thyroid gland.

Salmon, cod, and perch have a wide range of useful properties. Regular consumption of fish slows the aging process and improves potency. The highest amount of phosphorus is found in the gadoids fish: tuna, ling, haddock, hake, and cod. Meanwhile, perch fish, like pike and perch, are rich in protein and trace minerals. Sea bass is especially valuable, as it contains taurine and B vitamins. Among fish, flounder and mackerel are the holy grail of sexual potency. They should be included regularly in the diet of men who are over 50 because they stimulate libido.

Fish can also cause a burst of strength and energy because they contain omega-3 fatty acids, B vitamins (especially B12), as well as vitamins D, E, and A. Flounder even contains the amino acids threonine and glycine, as well as aspartic and glutamic acids. It also has zinc, potassium, sodium, magnesium, phosphorus, and calcium. Since the flesh of flounder lacks connective tissue, it is easier to digest and more readily absorbed by the body. This is part of what makes it such an effective aphrodisiac.

SALMON

Salmon flesh contains a large amount of melatonin, which is necessary for cellular rejuvenation. Salmon contains substances which improve brain function. Evidence shows that due to its unique composition, salmon can help male infertility because it improves blood circulation to the genital organs, increases potency, and improves erection. Legend tells us that like the salmon driving itself upstream to spawn, Aphrodite herself emerged from the sea foam.

The northern populations of the world, such as the Chukchi and the Inuits, have been eating pink salmon for centuries. Their excellent health and extreme physical endurance are legendary. The chemical composition of pink salmon contains almost the entire periodic table of elements. It has pyridoxine, which improves cellular metabolism, mood, and endurance. Salmon promotes a rush of blood to the genitals and normalizes erectile function. Likewise, it contains arginine, an amino acid required for the production of nitric oxide. The more nitrogen, the better quality erections for men and lubrication for women.

TROUT

In my opinion, Trout is a wonderful gift from the Goddess of Love. Like all fish, it is rich in Omega-3 fatty acids which benefits our heart, blood vessels, and hormones. Trout is good on its own, no matter how it is cooked. However, to get the most out of trout, it is best eaten with potherbs, vegetables, and certain spices. Trout is full of zinc and selenium, which promote the production of testosterone. Like salmon, it is rich in B vitamins and pyridoxine.

Trout can increase both your libido and your overall mood because it has such a remarkable taste.

HERRING

The herring is called a silver fish for two reasons. First, it gets its silver color from its shiny scales. Second, it brings silver coins into the pockets of fishermen who sell them, making up one-third of the entire world's fish commerce. A monument was erected to the man who presented the herring to the world: Jacob Boykelzoonom, a fisherman from the Dutch town Bierflint.

Today, fresh herring is considered a delicacy. Herring with caviar is called Rogner, while Milchner is herring with milt. Fish that haven't spawned are called Matjes or "virgin" herring. These are the most tender and tasty herring. Herring contains 20% fat, which accumulates in its muscles. It is equal in Omega-3 fatty acids to both eel and salmon.

Herring is unequaled in its Vitamin D content. You would need to eat an entire kilo of cheese, 15 eggs, or a kilo and half of a beef liver to get as much as a medium-sized fillet of herring. Herring also contains large amounts of iodine, potassium, vitamins B1, B6, B12, A, E, and selenium.

Herring was discovered to be an aphrodisiac in the 17th century, before the word "aphrodisiac" even existed. When examining patients, a French doctor noticed that the sexual desire of his patients who ate herring during a fast exceeded the sexual desire of those who did not. The men also had significantly higher semen quality. Scientists now know that herring cooked in sour cream improves erectile function, promoting a rush of blood to the genitals.

FLOUNDER

Flounder has exceptional aphrodisiac properties because it is rich in omega 3 fatty acids, niacin, pantothenic, aspartic and glutamic acids, pyridoxine, thiamine, riboflavin, and vitamins B12, D, E, and A. Trace minerals like selenium, zinc, phosphorus, sodium, potassium, calcium, copper, chromium, cobalt, and molybdenum are also present. And, at only 3% fat, its calorie content is only 83kcal per 100g.

Flounder protein is valuable because it has optimally balanced amino acids. They are quickly absorbed by the human body, creating a stimulating effect and increasing sexual desire. It is especially effective for older men and women. No wonder they call it "the love fish".

TUNA

Not many people know that the tuna is one of the fastest fish in the world. Physical activity is vital for tuna because their gills function only when they are in motion. It even remains in constant motion while it is asleep.

Regular consumption of tuna helps the whole body. It has plenty of vitamin D, omega 3 fatty acids, selenium, potassium, and sodium in ratios that are nearly perfect for humans. Tuna also does not lose its beneficial properties even after preserving. The French even call tuna "the marine veal," as its meat tastes more like beef than fish.

PIKE-PERCH (ZANDER)

Meat from this predatory fish is as nutritious as it is low in calories. In addition to 8 essential amino acids, pike-perch contains unsaturated omega-3 fatty acids, vitamins E, D, A, and the B group vitamins. It also contains minerals such as magnesium, potassium, phosphorus, cobalt, iodine, calcium, sulfur, and others. Meals created from pike-perch

51

increase endurance with sexual activity, and improve blood circulation to the genitals.

SOLE

Sole was once available only to the aristocracy. Rich in vitamin A, B1, B2, B3, and C, it is also a great supply of calcium, magnesium, sodium, potassium, phosphorus, and sulfur, as well as iron, zinc, iodine, copper, manganese, chromium, fluoride, molybdenum, cobalt, and nickel. Due to its essential fatty acid content of linoleic and arachidonic acids, as well as tryptophan, lysine, and methionine, it is a highly effective aphrodisiac.

Compared with flounder, which is a flatfish, sole has more of a delicate flavor. It is moderately fatty and yet contains almost no bones. You can feel free to experiment with using it in anything from the simplest to the most sophisticated of dishes. The French are considered the greatest sole connoisseurs in the world, and it shows in their cuisine. Italians love to cook sole in a dry white wine with strong Marsala. Spaniards like it fried and served with tomato sauce, pepper, almonds, and olive oil. Avoid hot spices and sauces, as they will drown out the delicate taste of the sole.

STURGEON

Sturgeon has tender white meat with amber fatty layers and black caviar. Only sturgeon has this particular kind of caviar, which is known as "black gold". This luxuriously delicate fish has been enjoyed by gourmets all over the world since ancient times. King Edward II of England (1284-1327), was so fond of sturgeon that he awarded it royal status. A representative of the sturgeon family, known as a sterlet, is considered to be a classic dish of Russian cuisine. Sterlet cooked in champagne was served for Nicholas II's coronation dinner. Prince Potemkin especially loved sterlet. It was not always easy to keep up with the demands of Catherine II, but the sterlet no doubt helped him manage to do so for many years!

Sturgeon contains a large amount of easily digestible proteins, vitamins A, B2, B3, C, D, E, and minerals such as sodium, phosphorus, chromium, nickel, and others. It also contains a lot of healthy fatty acids, making its calorie content rather high at 163.7kcal per 100g.

036 Salmon Pâté

INGREDIENTS

1 CAN OF SALMON
2 PACKS OF CREAM CHEESE
2.5 FL OZ (70 ML) OF KETCHUP
1 TSP OF LEMON JUICE
LETTUCE LEAVES FOR SERVING
MAYONNAISE FOR DECORATION
PARSLEY OR DILL

PREPARATION

Grind the salmon, cream cheese, ketchup, and lemon juice in a blender. Lay out the pâté in lightly oiled plastic wrap or a silicone mold. Refrigerate for 1 hour.

SERVING

Remove the pâté from the mold and lay it out on a platter covered with lettuce leaves. Decorate the dish with mayonnaise. Sprinkle with chopped parsley or place several dill sprigs atop it.

037 Red & White Appetizer

INGREDIENTS

10 SLICES OF SMOKED OR VACUUM-PACKED SALMON
5.5 OZ (150G) OF LOW-FAT COTTAGE CHEESE
2 TSP OF HORSERADISH
GROUND WHITE PEPPER
1 CUCUMBER FOR SERVING

PREPARATION

Lay the salmon out in overlapping rows on foil. Mix the cottage cheese, horseradish, and white pepper in a blender. Cover the fish with this mixture, and roll it up to enclose the filling. Wrap the roll in foil and refrigerate for 2-3 hours.

SERVING

Lay out the cucumber slices on a plate. Cut the salmon rolls into circular slices and place them atop the cucumber.

038 Smoked Salmon Ring Appetizer

INGREDIENTS

7 OZ (200G) OF SMOKED SALMON
½ LEEK STALK
1 TBSP OF CHOPPED DILL
4 LETTUCE LEAVES FOR SERVING
ZEST OF 1 LEMON

SAUCE:
2 TBSP OF MAYONNAISE
2 TBSP OF CREAM
1 TBSP OF LEMON JUICE
½ RED ONION
1 TSP OF CAPERS OR FINELY CHOPPED PICKLES
SALT & PEPPER

PREPARATION

Slice the salmon into small cubes. Add finely chopped leek and dill. To prepare the sauce: mix the mayonnaise with cream and lemon juice. Add onion, capers or finely chopped pickles. Season with salt and pepper. Cover the fish with this sauce and refrigerate for 30 minutes.

SERVING

Place the lettuce leaves on a plate. Place a culinary ring atop them and fill it with fish covered in sauce. Remove the ring and decorate the dish with capers and lemon zest.

039 Latin American Ceviche Appetizer

INGREDIENTS

17.5 OZ (500G) OF SALMON FILLET
1 HOT CHILI PEPPER
JUICE OF 2 LEMONS OR LIMES
1 RED ONION
1 BUNCH OF CILANTRO OR DILL
LEMON OR LIME ZEST

PREPARATION

Slice the fish fillets into cubes 2" (5cm) long. Cut the chili pepper in half crosswise. Cut the first half lengthwise and rub the mold with it. Remove the seeds from the second half. Cut it into rings and place them aside. Put the fish slices into the mold and cover them in citrus juice before mixing everything together. Refrigerate for a couple of hours.

SERVING

Place the marinated fish in a deep plate. Cover with thinly sliced red onion rings, chili pepper, chopped cilantro, dill, and finely chopped zest of lemon or lime.

040 Royal Salmon Bruschetta

INGREDIENTS

1 SMALL ONION
1 BELL PEPPER
1 OZ (30G) OF BUTTER
1 TBSP OF FLOUR
5 FL OZ (150 ML) OF MILK
1 HARDBOILED EGG YOLK
1 LOAF OF BREAD OR BAGUETTE
1 CAN OF SALMON
2 OZ (50G) OF PICKLED MUSHROOMS
SALT & GROUND PEPPER
SPRIGS OF PARSLEY OR CELERY FOR SERVING

PREPARATION

Finely chop the onion and bell pepper and fry them in butter until the mix becomes tender. Add the flour and start slowly pouring the milk while stirring constantly. Remove from heat and add boiled yolk to the mix.

SERVING

Slice the bread and dry the slices in the oven for 5 minutes. Place small pieces of salmon and pickled mushrooms on the toast. Pour the sauce over the fish. Decorate the dish with parsley or celery leaves.

041 Scottish Trout

INGREDIENTS

1 SMALL TROUT
SALT & PEPPER
1 TBSP OF MILK
1 OZ (25G) OF OAT FLOUR
1 TBSP OF VEGETABLE OIL
1 LEMON SLICE FOR SERVING
1 SPRIG OF PARSLEY

PREPARATION

Cut the trout into portions. Dip it into salted and peppered milk, and then bread the fish in oat flour. Fry the trout until it is cooked.

SERVING

Lay out the pieces of fried trout on a platter. Decorate the dish with a lemon slice and a sprig of parsley.

042 Nutty Trout

INGREDIENTS

4 FILLETS OF TROUT (WITH SKIN) WEIGHING 3.5 OZ
(100G) EACH
SALT & PEPPER
PARSLEY
2 ONIONS
1 TBSP OF MUSTARD
2 OZ (50G) OF BUTTER
JUICE OF 1 LEMON OR LIME
2 OZ (50G) OF ANY VARIETY OF CHOPPED NUTS
1 OZ (30G) THIN STRIPS OF BACON
LEMON OR LIME ZEST

PREPARATION

Make shallow cuts into the skin of fillets and season them
with salt and pepper. Lightly oil a sheet of aluminum foil.
Place two fillets on the foil, skin side down. Spread a mixture of chopped parsley, onion, mustard, half the butter,
and lemon or lime juice on top. Cover each fillet with another fillet, skin side up. Wrap up the foil. Bake the fish at
400°F (200°C) for 15-20 minutes.

SERVING

Put each fillet on a plate after removing from foil. Fry the
nuts and thin strips of bacon in the remaining butter for 5-
6 minutes. Lay everything out on the fish fillets. Decorate
the dish with lemon or lime zest.

043 Macedonian Trout

INGREDIENTS

1 TROUT
2.5 OZ (70G) OF PITTED PRUNES
3.5 FL OZ (100 ML) OF OLIVE OIL
1 TBSP OF WINE VINEGAR
4 CLOVES OF GARLIC
1 BUNCH OF PARSLEY
1 EGG
1 LEMON
SALT & PEPPER
2 FRESH CUCUMBERS FOR SERVING

PREPARATION

Parboil and scale the trout without damaging the skin. Steam the prunes for 5 minutes and stuff the trout with them. Add olive oil, vinegar, 2 cloves of crushed garlic, and finely chopped parsley to the saucepan. Place the trout on top of that and pour 13.5 fl oz (400 ml) of water over everything. Place the saucepan in an oven preheated to 350°F (180°C) for 20 minutes.

To prepare the sauce: whip the egg, grated garlic, parsley, and lemon juice in a blender. Refrigerate until thickened.

SERVING

Place the trout on a large oval platter. Draw patterns out of the lemon-garlic sauce around the fish using a pastry bag. Cut the cucumber into very thin diagonal circles and lay them out on the fish in the form of scales.

044 Trout in a Banana Coat

INGREDIENTS

1 SMALL TROUT
2 TBSP OF LEMON ZEST
5 CLOVES OF GARLIC
4 TBSP OF CORIANDER
1.5 FL OZ (40 ML) OF VEGETABLE OIL
SALT & GROUND BLACK PEPPER
SKINS OF 4 BANANAS
3.5 OZ (100G) OF BUTTER
1 TBSP OF GRATED GINGER ROOT
1 TBSP OF SOY SAUCE
1 LEMON FOR SERVING

PREPARATION

Wash the fish and scale it. Stuff it with a mixture of lemon zest, garlic, pepper, and coriander. Grease the fish with vegetable oil, salt, and pepper. Wrap up the fish in the banana skins. Bake it in the oven at 350°F (180°C) for 30 minutes.

To prepare the sauce: melt the butter and add ginger, garlic, and soy sauce to the saucepan.

SERVING

Lay out the fish on a large oval platter. Pour ginger sauce over it and sprinkle the dish with coriander. Decorate with lemon slices.

045 Trout in Caramel Sauce

INGREDIENTS

1 TROUT
4 FL OZ (125 ML) OF WATER
3 OZ (80G) OF SUGAR
3 TBSP OF FISH SAUCE
SALT & GROUND PEPPER
1 SMALL ONION
5-6 SMALL CHILI PEPPERS
1 SMALL GINGER ROOT

PREPARATION

Wash, scale, and gut the trout. Cut it into portions. Combine half the water with the sugar and put over high heat without stirring. Boil for 5 minutes. When the sugar begins to turn into caramel, remove the pan from heat. Add the remaining water, fish sauce, and salt. Put the pan back over the fire, reducing the heat to medium. Cut the onions into rings and add them to the caramel. Add the trout, peppers cut into strips, and chopped ginger. Stew the dish with the lid closed for 20 minutes. Flip the fish pieces and stew them for another 15 minutes.

SERVING

Put the trout pieces on individual dishes and generously cover with sauce. Place the chili peppers beside the fish.

046 "Who Likes It Hot?" Appetizer

INGREDIENTS

1 LARGE HERRING WITH MILT
4 HARDBOILED EGG YOLKS
1 TBSP OF MUSTARD
1.5 FL OZ (40 ML) OF OLIVE OR VEGETABLE OIL
1 LOAF OF WHITE BREAD
SPRIGS OF POTHERBS FOR SERVING

PREPARATION

Soak the herring in the milt. Remove the skin and bones. Cut the fish into slices. Knead hard-boiled egg yolks with mustard and milt. Gradually mix the vegetable oil into the egg mixture. Fry the slices of white bread in the oil. Cut the bread slices into circles. Lay out the egg mixture on fried bread and put 2 slices of herring on top of it. Bake in the oven at 350°F (180°C) for 5 minutes.

SERVING

Place a paper towel on a large platter and place the hot sandwiches on top. Decorate them with a sprig of dill, parsley, or celery.

047 Rollups Appetizer

INGREDIENTS

1 PICKLED CUCUMBER
1 CHOPPED ONION
A TSP OF GRAINED MUSTARD
5.5 OZ (150G) OF HERRING FILLETS
1 TBSP OF VINEGAR
A TSP OF VEGETABLE OIL
A TSP OF SUGAR
2 TBSP OF KABUL SAUCE (SEE BELOW)
4 TBSP OF REMOULADE SAUCE (SEE BELOW)

KABUL SAUCE:
26.5 OZ (750G) OF TOMATO PASTE
9 OZ (250G) OF COARSELY CHOPPED CARROTS
4.5 OZ (125G) OF CHOPPED ONION
2 HOT RED PEPPERS
4-5 ALLSPICE BERRIES
4 WHOLE CLOVES
34 FL OZ (1 LITER) OF 6% VINEGAR
34 FL OZ (1 LITER) OF MEAT BROTH

REMOULADE SAUCE:
3.5 OZ (100G) OF HERRING FILLET
1 PICKLED CUCUMBER
1 ONION
2 OZ (60G) OF CAPERS
3.5 FL OZ (100 ML) OF DRY WHITE WINE
20 FL OZ (600 ML) OF MAYONNAISE
2 OZ (60G) OF CHOPPED GREEN ONIONS
1 TBSP OF KABUL SAUCE
SALT & GROUND BLACK PEPPER

PREPARATION

To prepare the Kabul sauce: put tomato paste, coarsely chopped carrots, onion, red chili peppers, allspice, clove, vinegar, and meat broth into the saucepan. Boil it on low heat until the vegetables become soft. Strain through a sieve and boil until you get a syrupy liquid. Pour the sauce into jars and refrigerate for 15 minutes.

To prepare the Remoulade sauce: finely chop the herring, pickled cucumber, onion, and capers. Combine all the ingredients. Add dry wine, mayonnaise, finely chopped spring onions, and Kabul sauce. Season the sauce with salt and pepper to your taste.

Put slices of pickled cucumber, finely chopped onion, and grained mustard on the herring fillets and roll them up. Prepare the marinade by dissolving vinegar and oil in a small amount of water. Fasten the rolls with a wooden skewer and cover them with marinade for 2-3 days.

SERVING

When serving, sprinkle the herring rolls with Remoulade sauce and decorate them with a sprig of parsley.

048 Swedish Glazier Herring

INGREDIENTS

8 FAT HERRINGS
7 OZ (200G) OF ONION
5.5 OZ (150G) OF CARROTS
1 OZ (30G) OF HORSERADISH
1 TBSP OF GROUND RED PEPPER
10 PEPPERCORNS
10 WHOLE BAY LEAVES
1 OZ (30G) OF MUSTARD
GINGER TO TASTE
13.5 FL OZ (400 ML) OF WATER
10 FL OZ (300 ML) OF VINEGAR
10 OZ (300G) OF POWDERED SUGAR
FEATHERS OF SPRING ONIONS FOR SERVING

PREPARATION

Scale the herring. Soak it in water for 12 hours. You will need to change the water several times until it becomes transparent. Cut the fish into fillets. Add sliced onions, carrots, horseradish, and spices. Boil water with vinegar and sugar. Let it cool and pour it over the herring. Refrigerate for 5 days.

SERVING

Slice the herring into portions. Lay it out in the form of a pigtail on a herring dish, and decorate the dish with spring onions.

049 Herring Bird Nests

INGREDIENTS

3.5 OZ (100G) OF HERRING FILLET
½ ONION
1 TBSP (20G) OF CAPERS OR PICKLES
2 HARDBOILED EGG YOLKS
LETTUCE LEAVES FOR SERVING

PREPARATION

Finely chop the herring fillets. Add chopped onion, capers, and pickles. Mix well and shape into balls. Insert an egg yolk into each to form a nest.

SERVING

Serve the dish on lettuce leaves.

050 Norwegian Herring Salad

INGREDIENTS

3.5 OZ (100G) OF LIGHTLY SALTED HERRING FILLET
½ SMALL ONION
1 TSP OF VEGETABLE OIL
1 EGG
1 TBSP OF 15% VINEGAR
½ TSP OF SUGAR
½ TSP OF MUSTARD
PARSLEY
1 HARDBOILED EGG FOR SERVING

PREPARATION

Cut the herring fillet into cubes. Fry finely chopped onion in vegetable oil. Whip up the egg with vinegar. Pour the mixture over the onions and heat it until the eggs start curdling. Season everything with sugar and mustard before letting it cool.

SERVING

Pour the sauce on a plate and place the fillets on top. Decorate the dish with parsley and slices of hard-boiled egg.

051 Love Boat Appetizer

INGREDIENTS

2 WHOLE FLOUNDERS
4 TOMATOES
7 OZ (200G) OF ANY KIND OF HARD CHEESE
SALT & GROUND PEPPER
1 BUNCH OF SPRING ONIONS
THYME OR OREGANO FOR SERVING

PREPARATION

Wash the fish and dry it with a paper towel. Make cuts along the backbone, forming little pockets. Fill these pockets with a mixture of finely chopped tomatoes and cheese. Season the fish with salt and pepper, roll it in flour, and fry it on both sides for 2 minutes each. Wrap each fish in foil, forming a foil boat and leaving the top of the boat open. Bake at 350°F (180°C) for 20 minutes.

SERVING

Place 1 boat on each serving plate. Sprinkle it with spring onions and thyme or oregano.

052 Stuffed Flounder

INGREDIENTS

2 MEDIUM-SIZED FLOUNDERS
SALT & GROUND BLACK PEPPER
1 LEMON
5.5 OZ (150G) OF BOILED & SHELLED SHRIMP
5.5 OZ (150G) OF BLUE CHEESE OR ANY HARD CHEESE
2 FL OZ (50 ML) OF HEAVY CREAM
1 BUNCH OF DILL
LETTUCE LEAVES
A HANDFUL OF SESAME SEEDS
1 LEMON SLICE FOR SERVING

PREPARATION

Scale the fish, and season it with salt and pepper. Sprinkle with lemon juice inside and out.

To prepare the stuffing, clean the boiled shrimp and knead the cheese with a fork (if you have a hard cheese, grate it). Whip the heavy cream and cheese into a mixture, adding dill, shrimp, and lemon zest. Season it with salt and pepper. Cut the flounder with a sharp knife along the backbone and fill it with the stuffing. Oil the fish and wrap it in foil. Bake at 350°F (180°C) for 15 minutes. Unwrap the foil and continue baking for 5 additional minutes.

SERVING

Place the lettuce on a plate. Lay out the fish without foil and sprinkle it with sesame seeds. Put a slice of lemon beside the fish.

053 Bloody Josephine Baked Flounder

INGREDIENTS

10 OZ (300G) OF PEELED TOMATOES
3.5 OZ (100G) OF BUTTER
4 FLOUNDER FILLETS
BREADCRUMBS
DRIED BASIL & ITALIAN POTHERBS
1 SPRIG OF ROSEMARY OR THYME
SEVERAL LEAVES OF FRESH GREEN & PURPLE BASIL
FOR SERVING

PREPARATION

Smash the tomatoes in a blender and strain them to remove the juice. Melt the butter in a saucepan. Add the tomatoes and season them with salt and pepper. Stew the tomatoes over low heat for 25 minutes. Roll the flounder fillets in flour and lightly fry them.

Place fillets in a refractory mold and cover them with tomato-cream sauce. Sprinkle with breadcrumbs mixed with the dry potherbs. Place rosemary sprigs between the fillets. Season the fish with salt and pepper. Bake at 375°F (190°C) until the crust becomes golden (approx. 30 minutes).

SERVING

Put 2 flounder fillets on plates. Generously pour tomato-cream sauce over the fish and place basil leaves on top.

054 Rosy Flounder Rolls

INGREDIENTS

4 PIECES OF FLOUNDER FILLETS
1 LEMON
FISH SPICES (SUCH AS ROSEMARY, BASIL, OREGANO, DILL, OR FENNEL)
4 THIN SLICES OF HAM
VEGETABLE OIL FOR FRYING
1 ONION
1 CAN OF TOMATOES IN THEIR OWN JUICE
TOMATO SAUCE
LETTUCE LEAVES FOR SERVING
BASIL OR PARSLEY

PREPARATION

Wash the fillets and dry them with a paper towel. Sprinkle with lemon juice and season with fish spices and lemon zest. Wrap the ham slices around the fish. Lightly drizzle the rolls with oil. Cook them in a double boiler for 20 minutes. Meanwhile, prepare the sauce by frying finely chopped onion in vegetable oil. Add tomatoes and tomato sauce, as well as the spices. Boil everything for a few minutes.

Before serving, fry the rolls in vegetable oil until the ham becomes golden.

SERVING

Place the lettuce leaves on serving plates and put 2 rolls on top. Drizzle them with the sauce. Sprinkle the dish with basil or parsley.

055 Flounder Under Bread Crust

INGREDIENTS

4 LARGE TOMATOES
3.5 OZ (100G) OF BUTTER
FISH SPICES (SUCH AS ROSEMARY, BASIL, OREGANO, DILL, OR FENNEL)
SALT
4 FLOUNDER FILLETS
BASIL
BREADCRUMBS
JUICE OF ½ LEMON
2 LEMON SLICES FOR SERVING

PREPARATION

Pour boiling water over tomatoes. Peel and strain through a sieve. Melt butter in a saucepan. Add tomatoes, fish spices, and salt. Cook mix on low heat for 20 minutes, occasionally stirring. Wash the flounder fillets, dry them with paper towels, roll the fish in flour, and fry. Put the fried fillets into a refractory mold and pour the tomato sauce over them. Season with potherbs and basil, and generously sprinkle the fish with breadcrumbs. Bake in the oven at 350°F (180°C) until the flounder becomes golden brown.

SERVING

Place the contents of the mold on 1 large platter. Sprinkle the dish with basil again and drizzle it with lemon juice. Lay out the lemon slices on the plate diagonally.

056 Tuna Salad in Avocado Boats

INGREDIENTS

1 LARGE AVOCADO
2 BOILED EGGS
1 RED ONION
1 CAN OF TUNA
3.5 FL OZ (100 ML) OF SOUR CREAM
SALT & PEPPER
SEVERAL SPRING ONIONS FOR SERVING

PREPARATION

Cut the avocado in half and remove the pit. Remove the pulp of the avocado with a dessert spoon and finely chop it, setting the skin aside. Chop the eggs and red onion. Drain the oil from the tuna can and mash the tuna meat with a fork. Mix all the ingredients and dress them with sour cream. Season the salad with salt and pepper to your taste.

SERVING

Stuff avocado skins with salad. Decorate with spring onions.

057 Ensalada Mediterranea

INGREDIENTS

2 TOMATOES
1 ONION
1 CARROT
4 BOILED QUAIL EGGS
1 CAN OF TUNA
1 BUNCH OF LETTUCE
1 CAN OF CORN
7 OZ (200G) OF BLACK OR GREEN OLIVES
SALT & COARSELY GROUND PEPPER

SAUCE:
3.5 FL OZ (100 ML) OF OLIVE OIL
2 TBSP OF WINE VINEGAR
½ TBSP OF MUSTARD

PREPARATION

Slice the tomatoes. Cut the onion and carrot into strips and cut the eggs into halves. Drain the oil from the tuna can and mash the tuna meat with a fork. To prepare the sauce: mix olive oil, vinegar, and mustard in a blender.

SERVING

Put the lettuce leaves onto 2 plates. Place the tomatoes, quail eggs, onions, carrots, tuna, corn and olives on top. Use the sauce as a dressing. Season the salad with salt and pepper.

058 Spanish Themed Tuna Salad

INGREDIENTS

1 RED ONION
3.5 OZ (100G) OF BLUE CHEESE
1 CAN OF TUNA
1 EAR OF CORN
1 CAN OF OLIVES
SEVERAL FRESH BASIL LEAVES FOR SERVING

SAUCE:
2.5 FL OZ (75 ML) OF OLIVE OIL
1 TBSP OF BALSAMIC VINEGAR
1 TBSP OF LEMON JUICE

PREPARATION

Finely chop the onion. Crumble the cheese and mash the tuna with a fork. Mix the corn, onion, tuna, cheese, and olives. To prepare the sauce: mix all the ingredients with a whisk.

SERVING

Place the salad on a round white dish. Dress it with the sauce and decorate with basil leaves.

059 Pistachio Breaded Tuna

INGREDIENTS

20 OZ (600G) OF FRESH TUNA
1 TBSP OF SOY SAUCE
2.5 FL OZ (75 ML) OF OLIVE OIL
1 OZ (30G) OF DRIED TOMATOES
2 OZ (50G) OF PISTACHIOS
1 TBSP OF WHITE BREADCRUMBS
1 TBSP OF SESAME SEEDS
4 LARGE LETTUCE LEAVES FOR SERVING
1 CAN OF RED BEANS FOR GARNISH

PREPARATION

Cut the tuna meat into small pieces less than 1" (3cm) long. Sprinkle the pieces with soy sauce and 1 tablespoon of olive oil. Finely chop the dried tomatoes. Grind the pistachios in a blender. Mix the breadcrumbs, tomatoes, pistachios, and sesame seeds. Roll the tuna in the breadcrumb mixture. Fry it in the remaining olive oil until it is done.

SERVING

Place 2 large lettuce leaves on 2 serving plates. Put the pistachio breaded tuna on 1 leaf and the canned red beans on the other.

060 Cheese Tempura Tuna with Sesame seeds

INGREDIENTS

14 OZ (400G) OF TUNA FILLET
2 FL OZ (60 ML) OF SOY SAUCE
1 OZ (25G) OF HONEY
2 TSP OF LEMON JUICE
2.5 FL OZ (75 ML) OF VEGETABLE OIL
2 EGGS
9 OZ (250G) OF FETA CHEESE
1 TBSP OF GRATED PARMESAN CHEESE
1 TBSP OF FLOUR

BREADING:
1.5 OZ (40G) OF SESAME SEEDS
1 TBSP OF CUMIN

PREPARATION

Cut tuna into steaks. Mix soy sauce, honey or pomegranate sauce, lemon juice, and vegetable oil. Marinade fish for 20 minutes, periodically flipping. Prepare tempura by mixing eggs, feta and parmesan cheese, and flour. To make breading, mix sesame seeds and cumin. Drain steaks and cover them with tempura. Sprinkle the fish with breading on both sides. Fry for 4 minutes on each side. Roast the string beans in a mixture of vegetable oil and soy sauce.

SERVING

Place steaks on large round plates with mint. Lay the string beans to the side. Sprinkle the string beans with any berries.

79

061 Cod Fillet with Coffee Plume in a Velvet Sauce

INGREDIENTS

17.5 OZ (500G) OF COD FILLET
GROUND BLACK PEPPER
1 OZ (30G) OF VEGETABLE OIL
2 FL OZ (50G) OF BUTTER
1 TBSP OF COFFEE BEANS
1 ORANGE
1 TSP OF BROWN SUGAR
2 FL OZ (50 ML) OF 33% FAT CREAM
1 OZ (30G) OF BITTER DARK CHOCOLATE
1 TBSP OF SOY SAUCE

PREPARATION

Wash cod fillets and dry them with a paper towel. Rub the fish with pepper and grease it with vegetable oil. Fry the cod in a frying pan to a golden color. Grease each side of the fillets with softened butter and put several coffee beans on the fillets. Put the fillets on parchment paper and wrap them carefully. Bake for 12 minutes at 400°F (200°C).

To prepare sauce: squeeze juice from the orange and add brown sugar. Boil in a saucepan for 10 minutes until thickened. Add cream and bitter dark chocolate. Stir everything and add soy sauce to the saucepan. Remove from heat.

SERVING

Pour the sauce into 2 dishes and put the cod fillets on top.

062 Spicy & Nutty Breaded Cod

INGREDIENTS

A SPRIG OF ROSEMARY
2 FL OZ (50 ML) OF VEGETABLE BROTH
2 CLOVES OF GARLIC
JUICE OF ½ LEMON
5.5 OZ (150G) OF COD FILLET
SALT & BLACK OR LEMON PEPPER
1 EGG
2 OZ (50G) OF BREADCRUMBS
2 OZ (50G) OF ANY VARIETY OF CHOPPED NUTS
3 TBSP OF OLIVE OIL
1 TSP OF CAPERS
PARSLEY

PREPARATION

Wash a sprig of rosemary and add it to the vegetable broth. Add chopped garlic and lemon juice. Place this fragrant mixture on a plate where the cod will be served.

Wash the cod and cut it into portions. Season with salt and pepper and sprinkle with lemon juice. Roll the fish first in the egg, and then breadcrumbs and nuts. Fry the cod in hot oil for 4-5 minutes on each side.

SERVING

Place the fried fish on the garlic mixture. Make a spicy mixture from capers, chopped parsley, and lemon juice and place it on each slice of the cod.

063 Cod Salad on a Vegetable Bed

INGREDIENTS

7 OZ (200G) OF COD
1 TBSP OF LEMON JUICE
A PINCH OF OREGANO
1 APPLE
1 CARROT
1 CUCUMBER
2 TOMATOES
SALT & GROUND BLACK PEPPER
3 TBSP OF SOY SAUCE
LETTUCE LEAVES FOR SERVING
1 CELERY STALK FOR GARNISH

PREPARATION

Boil the cod fillet and cut it into small pieces. Sprinkle with lemon juice and season with oregano. Refrigerate until ready to serve. Peel an apple and a carrot and cut them into strips. Slice the cucumber and tomatoes into half circles. Mix the vegetables. Season them with salt and pepper and pour the soy sauce over them. Gently mix everything once more.

SERVING

Put lettuce leaves on 2 plates and lay the vegetables on top in a bed. Lay out the pieces of cod over the vegetable bed. Sprinkle the salad with chopped celery and pepper.

064 Baked Cod with Cheese Sauce

INGREDIENTS

2 FL OZ (60 ML) OF SOUR CREAM
2 OZ (50G) OF GRATED PARMESAN CHEESE
2 CLOVES OF GARLIC
1 BUNCH OF PARSLEY
1 SMALL BUNCH OF BASIL
4 PORTIONED PIECES OF COD
SEA SALT & BLACK PEPPER
2 LEMON SLICES FOR SERVING

PREPARATION

Mix the sour cream and grated cheese. Add chopped garlic and potherbs. Wash the cod pieces and dry them with paper towels. Season with salt. Preheat the oven to 450°F (230°C). Cover the baking tray with baking paper and put the cod pieces, evenly covered with sour cream cheese sauce, on top. Bake for 10 minutes or until the fish begins to flake. Switch the oven to grill mode and bake to a golden color.

SERVING

Place 2 pieces of fish per portion, with a lemon slice beside the fish.

065 Cod with Pears

INGREDIENTS

2 COD FILLETS WEIGHING 7 OZ (200G) EACH
JUICE OF ½ LEMON
ROSEMARY
THYME
SEA SALT & WHITE PEPPER
2 PEARS
1.5 OZ (40G) OF PITTED PRUNES
1 TBSP OF VEGETABLE OIL
1 TSP OF CHOPPED DILL FOR SERVING

PREPARATION

Marinate the cod fillets in a mixture of lemon juice, rosemary, and thyme for 10 minutes. Cut the pears and prunes into small cubes. Place a spoonful on each fillet and roll them up. Fasten the rolls with wooden skewers. Bake the dish for 20 minutes at 300°F (150°C) in a preheated oven.

SERVING

Place a roll on each plate. Sprinkle with chopped potherbs.

066 Bakonian Pike-Perch Fillet

INGREDIENTS

10 OZ (300G) OF SKINLESS PIKE-PERCH FILLET
1 TBSP OF BUTTER
½ ONION
3.5 OZ (100G) OF MUSHROOMS
RED PEPPER TO TASTE
5 FL OZ (150 ML) OF FISH BROTH
1 FL OZ (40 ML) OF SOUR CREAM
1 TBSP OF FLOUR
SALT
1 GREEN BELL PEPPER
CELERY OR PARSLEY FOR SERVING

PREPARATION

Cut the fish into portions and place them in a greased sauce-pan. Prepare the sauce by sautéing chopped onions in butter, then add mushrooms and red pepper and sauté until tender. Pour fish broth and sour cream mixed with flour over the fish. Bake in the oven at 350°F (180°C) for 20 minutes until cooked.

SERVING

Decorate the dish with thin slices of green bell pepper and celery or parsley.

067 Pike-Perch Orly

INGREDIENTS

7 OZ (200G) OF SKINLESS PIKE-PERCH FILLET
2 TBSP OF VEGETABLE OIL
1 TSP OF LEMON JUICE
SALT & GROUND BLACK PEPPER
1 EGG
1.5 OZ (40G) OF FLOUR
1 FL OZ (40 ML) OF BEER
1 LEMON SLICE & 1 SPRIG OF PARSLEY FOR SERVING
1 FL OZ (30 ML) OF TOMATO SAUCE
70G OF MAYONNAISE

PREPARATION

Put the pike-perch fillets in a bowl with vegetable oil and lemon juice. Sprinkle with salt, pepper, and chopped parsley. Marinate the fish for 20 minutes. Dip the fish pieces into a batter made from eggs, flour, and beer. Deep fry the battered fish.

SERVING

Lay the fillets out in the form of a pyramid. Decorate with a lemon slice and a sprig of parsley. Mix tomato sauce with mayonnaise and serve it separately from the fish.

068 Pike-Perch with Vanilla

INGREDIENTS

1 VANILLA BEAN
1 CARROT
1 ZUCCHINI
½ GREEN APPLE
1 STICK OF BUTTER
1 SPRIG OF BASIL
17.5 OZ (500G) OF PIKE-PERCH FILLETS

PREPARATION

Cut the vanilla bean in half and place it in warm butter. Chop the vegetables and apple into strips and fry them in oil. Add chopped basil. Lay out the vegetables on a serving dish and set aside. Pan fry the pike-perch fillets in the vanilla butter on the stove until it forms a crust. Then add more butter. Bake the fish in the oven at 350°F (180°C) for 5 minutes.

SERVING

Bring out the prepared serving dish of chopped vegetables. Place the baked pike-perch fillet and a piece of vanilla on top.

069 Appetizing Pike-Perch

INGREDIENTS

2 MEDIUM-SIZED PIKE-PERCH
2 CARROTS
1 ONION
1 CAN OF COD LIVER
3.5 OZ (100G) OF BREADCRUMBS
3.5 FL OZ (100 ML) OF MAYONNAISE
SALT & PEPPER
1 TBSP OF MOZZARELLA CHEESE
LETTUCE LEAVES
2 LEMON SLICES FOR SERVING
2 SPRIGS OF DILL

PREPARATION

Scale, gut, and wash fish. Leave a carrot to stew for 25 minutes and grate another. Sauté the onion and grated carrot in vegetable oil. Let cool and add chopped cod liver, breadcrumbs, and mayonnaise. Season with salt and pepper. Stuff both fish, and sew up the belly with thread. Make cuts along the backbone and put cheese slices inside. Cover the pike-perch with mayonnaise and sprinkle it with grated cheese. Bake the fish at 350°F (180°C) to a golden crust.

SERVING

Lay out lettuce leaves on 2 plates and put baked fish on top. Put a slice of lemon and a sprig of dill right beside each.

070 Mexican Style Pike-Perch

INGREDIENTS

2 PIKE-PERCH FILLETS
2 FL OZ (50 ML) OF CREAM
2 FL OZ (70 ML) OF MILK
1 FL OZ (30 ML) OF FISH BROTH
2 FL OZ (50 ML) OF DRY WHITE WINE
2 OZ (50G) OF HARD CHEESE
JUICE OF 1 LEMON
FISH SPICES (ROSEMARY, BASIL, OREGANO, OR DILL)
1 CUP OF RAW RICE
CILANTRO
SEVERAL SPRING ONIONS
PARSLEY
1 HOT PICKLED PEPPER

PREPARATION

Fry the fish fillets in a pan. To prepare the sauce: mix cream, milk, fish broth, wine, grated cheese, and lemon juice in a saucepan. Season the sauce with salt and spices to your taste. Cook until the sauce is thickened. Pour the sauce over the fillets and stew the fish for 5 more minutes.

Boil the rice until it is cooked. Add chopped cilantro, spring onions, parsley, hot pickled pepper, and olive oil. This combination of ingredients will give a green color to the rice.

SERVING

Lay out the fillets on plates and garnish with green rice.

071 Sole Rolls à la Saint-Damber

INGREDIENTS

2 SOLE FILLETS
JUICE OF 1 LEMON
2 FL OZ (50 ML) OF DRY WHITE WINE
1 LEMON SLICE
A SPRIG OF PARSLEY FOR SERVING

BEURRE BLANC SAUCE (WHITE BUTTERY SAUCE):
3.5 FL OZ (100 ML) OF DRY WHITE WINE
1 FL OZ (40 ML) OF WINE VINEGAR
2 TBSP OF FINELY CHOPPED SHALLOT
2 FL OZ (50 ML) OF CREAM
SALT & WHITE PEPPER
7 OZ (200G) OF BUTTER

PREPARATION

Make rolls out of sole fillets and fasten with toothpicks or wooden skewers. Sprinkle the rolls with lemon juice and boil in a mixture of water and dry wine, stirring frequently.

To prepare sauce: bring dry white wine to a boil. Add wine vinegar and finely chopped shallots. Boil for 5 minutes. Add cream and season with salt and white pepper. Let boil for 1 minute. Add butter to sauce. Boil for 5 minutes. Let cool.

SERVING

Lay out fish roll on a plate and pour the sauce over it. Place a lemon slice and a sprig of parsley right beside the roll.

072 Baked Sole Diane

INGREDIENTS

2 SMALL SOLE FILLETS
3.5 FL OZ (100 ML) OF DRY WHITE WINE
7 FL OZ (200 ML) OF WHITE SAUCE
3.5 OZ (100G) OF WHITE SEEDLESS GRAPES FOR
SERVING

WHITE SAUCE:
2 TBSP OF BUTTER
1 TBSP OF FLOUR
8 FL OZ (250 ML) OF MILK
SALT & PEPPER
1 GRATED NUTMEG

PREPARATION

Simmer the sole in white wine. Remove from pan and put
in a baking dish. Pour white sauce over it. Bake in the oven
at 350°F (180°C) for 20-25 minutes.

To prepare the sauce: melt the butter in a pan. Fry flour in
the pan and add milk. Stir the sauce constantly and bring it
to a boil. Season with salt and pepper to your taste. Add
nutmeg. If lumps form, mix in a blender or strain through a
sieve.

SERVING

Place baked sole on a plate. Lay out the white grapes in a
single line in the center along the fillets. Spread the rest of
the grapes randomly on the plate.

073 Sole with Light Shrimp

INGREDIENTS

3.5 FL OZ (100 ML) OF DRY WHITE WINE
3.5 OZ (100G) OF SHRIMP
SPRING ONIONS
1 SOLE FILLET
JUICE OF ½ LEMON
SALT & PEPPER
2 BELL PEPPERS OF DIFFERENT COLORS

PREPARATION

Pour the dry wine into a pan over low heat. Add peeled shrimp, chopped onion, and sole fillet. Cut the sole fillet into slices and sprinkle them with lemon juice. Fry until cooked throughout.

SERVING

Place the content of the pan onto a large platter. Lay out the pepper rings beside the fish.

074 Sole on Eggplant under Aioli

INGREDIENTS

3 RED BELL PEPPERS
2 FL OZ (50 ML) OF VEGETABLE OIL
1 LARGE EGGPLANT
28 OZ (800G) OF SOLE FILLETS
2 TBSP OF BUTTER
SALT & PEPPER
2 SPRIGS OF DILL & PARSLEY
4 BAGUETTE SLICES FOR SERVING

AIOLI SAUCE:
4 CLOVES OF GARLIC
2 RAW EGG YOLKS
1 TBSP OF LEMON JUICE
SALT
8.5 FL OZ (250 ML) OF OLIVE OIL

PREPARATION

Wash peppers. Cut them into halves, removing the insides
and seeds. Lay the peppers out on a greased baking pan with
the skin up. Lightly oil them. Bake at 400°F (200°C) for 15-
20 minutes. Move them into a glass bowl covered with cling
film and set aside. After cooling, peel and purée 2 of the
peppers in a blender. Save 1 pepper for serving.

Cut the eggplant (with skin) into circles ½" (1cm) thick.
Season them with salt and set aside for 20 minutes to remove bitterness. Wash and dry the eggplant with a paper

towel. Grease with vegetable oil and bake in the oven at 400°F (200°C) for 15 minutes until softened.

Cut the fish into portioned pieces. Fry them in butter until golden brown (3-4 minutes).

To prepare the aioli sauce: chop the garlic. Whip the egg yolks with lemon juice and salt. Slowly pour in a thin stream of olive oil without turning off the mixer. Keep whipping until the sauce becomes thick.

Add the roasted pepper purée and finely chopped parsley or dill. Cover the baguette slices with olive oil and put them into the oven for 3 minutes. Turn it off and leave the bread in the oven for another 3 minutes. Rub with garlic.

SERVING

Put 2 slices of eggplant on a large dish. Lay out a few strips of roasted red pepper on the eggplant and place fried sole pieces on top. Put 2 slices of bread right beside the fish.

075 Vertigo Sole in Champagne Sauce

INGREDIENTS

2 SOLE FILLETS WEIGHING 17.5 OZ (500G) EACH
1 TBSP OF LEMON JUICE
SEA SALT & FRESHLY GROUND BLACK PEPPER
1 TSP OF CHOPPED PARSLEY & CELERY
2 SPRIGS OF CHERVIL OR FENNEL FOR SERVING

SAUCE:
2 OZ (50G) OF BUTTER
1 SHALLOT
10 OZ (300G) OF RAW SHRIMP
10 FL OZ (300 ML) OF BRUT CHAMPAGNE
10 FL OZ (100 ML) OF HEAVY CREAM
SALT & PEPPER TO TASTE

PREPARATION

Rinse fillets and dry with a paper towel. Drizzle with lemon juice, then season with salt and pepper. Sprinkle with chopped parsley and celery. Steam for 10 minutes.

To prepare sauce: melt the butter in a saucepan and fry the shallots until soft. Add shrimp, pour champagne, and bring everything to a boil. Add the cream and simmer the sauce, but do not let it boil. Season the sauce with salt and pepper.

SERVING

Put fillets on pre-warmed plates. Pour over with champagne sauce. Decorate with a sprig of chervil or fennel.

076 Sturgeon Satsivi

INGREDIENTS

14 OZ (400G) OF BELUGA OR STELLATE STURGEON
SALT & GROUND BLACK PEPPER
SEVERAL BAY LEAVES
3 CLOVES OF GARLIC
1 CUP OF CRUSHED WALNUTS
1 HOT PEPPER
1 TSP OF CORIANDER SEEDS
3 ONIONS
CINNAMON
CLOVES
3.5 FL OZ (100 ML) OF WINE VINEGAR
CHOPPED CORIANDER OR PARSLEY
SEVERAL LEMON SLICES FOR SERVING

PREPARATION

Cut fish into portions and place in boiling salted water. Remove foam. Add a bay leaf and allspice. Cook for 30 minutes. Lay out fish on a plate. Combine crushed garlic with nuts, hot pepper, and coriander seeds, then dilute this mix with fish broth and fat from cooking. Add finely chopped onion. Boil sauce for 10 minutes on low heat. Add the cinnamon, cloves, pepper, and vinegar. Cook for 10 minutes more. Pour the hot sauce over the fish and let cool.

SERVING

This dish is especially suitable for a special occasion. It should be served on a decorative plate. Decorate the dish with finely chopped coriander or parsley, alternating with slices of lemon along the circumference of the plate.

077 Sturgeon under Lyon Sauce

INGREDIENTS

1 STURGEON WEIGHING APPROX. 4.5LBS (2KG)
SALT & WHITE PEPPER
1 LEMON
SEVERAL SPRIGS OF PARSLEY
2 FL OZ (50 ML) OF DRY WHITE WINE
1 TOMATO
1 LEMON
DILL
OLIVES FOR SERVING

LYON SAUCE:
1 OZ (30G) OF BUTTER
2 TBSP OF FLOUR
3.5 FL OZ (100 ML) OF FISH BROTH
1 LEEK
1 BUNCH OF PARSLEY
1 BUNCH OF DILL
2 FL OZ (50 ML) OF DRY WHITE WINE
1 EGG YOLK

PREPARATION

To prepare the fish: gently gut the sturgeon without damaging the gallbladder and remove the gills. Wash it under running water. Dry with a paper towel. Thoroughly rub the fish with salt and set aside for 5 minutes. Wash, dry, and rub the fish with salt and pepper once more. Cut the lemon into thick circles. Wrap the lemon circles in parsley and place inside the fish belly.

Cover the baking pan with foil and grease it with vegetable oil. Lay out the stuffed fish. Pour it over with dry wine and carefully wrap the fish in foil. Bake at 400°F (200°C) for 15 minutes. Unwrap the foil and put it into the oven for another 25 minutes.

To prepare the Lyon sauce: melt half the butter in a saucepan. Add flour and fish broth. Mix everything. Separately, fry the leeks and potherbs in a mixture of vegetable oil and butter. Add wine and let stew for another 5 minutes. Combine both mixtures, and carefully add foamy whipped egg yolk. Warm everything and remove from heat. Strain the mass through a sieve. Let it cool and add remaining butter.

SERVING

Put the sturgeon on a large and elegant oblong dish. Place tomato and lemon circles on both sides of the plate. Decorate the dish with olives and cover in sauce.

078 Searing Moment Canapés

INGREDIENTS

1 TBSP OF MAYONNAISE
1 TSP OF GRATED HORSERADISH
4 SLICES OF TRIANGULAR WHITE BREAD
4 SLICES OF BOILED STURGEON
24 OLIVES FOR SERVING
4 PIECES OF BLACK OLIVES FOR CANAPÉS
1 MARINATED RED HOT PEPPER

PREPARATION

Mix mayonnaise with grated horseradish. Cover the bread with this mix and put a piece of fish on each slice of bread.

SERVING

Place 2 canapés spaced apart on 2 plates. Lay out a trail of olives between them. Place a black olive and a strip of red hot pepper on each canapé.

079 Royal Sturgeon

INGREDIENTS

1 MEDIUM-SIZED STURGEON
3.5 FL OZ (100 ML) OF WHITE WINE OR CHAMPAGNE
SALT & PEPPER
2 FL OZ (50 ML) OF SOUR CREAM & MAYONNAISE
1 CAN OF PITTED OLIVES
15 PIECES OF PINK SALMON
SEVERAL BOILED & PEELED QUAIL EGGS
2 ONIONS WORTH OF PICKLED ONION RINGS
POTHERBS
1 TBSP OF VEGETABLE OIL
MAYONNAISE
2 OZ (50G) OF RED CAVIAR
1 BUNCH OF DILL FOR SERVING

PREPARATION

Wash the sturgeon. Remove its insides and the chord. Cut off its spikes with scissors. Marinate the fish for 15 minutes in wine or champagne. Rub it with salt and pepper. Cover the sturgeon with a mix of sour cream and mayonnaise. Stuff it with olives, slices of salmon, quail eggs, pickled onions, and potherbs. Grease the baking pan with vegetable oil. Bake the fish until it is cooked.

SERVING

Place the portioned fish on a large oval dish. Decorate each piece with a pattern of mayonnaise and place red caviar inside it. Spread chopped dill along the perimeter of the fish.

080 Rockefeller Sturgeon

INGREDIENTS

1 STURGEON WEIGHING APPROX. 3.5LBS (1.5KG)
1 ONION
1 CARROT
BAY LEAF
ALLSPICE
3 EGGS
SALT
2 STALE BREAD LOAVES
3.5 FL OZ (100 ML) OF VEGETABLE OIL
LETTUCE LEAVES
4 CANS OF WHOLE CORN
LEMON SLICES FOR SERVING
BLACK OLIVES

SAUCE:
10 OZ (300G) OF MAYONNAISE
1 HORSERADISH ROOT
3 TBSP OF SUGAR
SALT

PREPARATION

Boil water in a saucepan. Put the fish in the water and leave it for 5 minutes before removing. Clear the spikes from the fish skin. Bring the water back to a boil. Add the whole onion and carrots to the water, followed by the bay leaf and allspice to create vegetable broth. Put the fish in the broth and reduce the heat. Let stew until the fish becomes tender. Cool the fish in the broth. Meanwhile, grind the eggs with salt. Crush stale white bread into crumbs with a blender. Remove the fish from the broth. Dry it and cut into portions.

Dip each piece of the fish into the egg and then into the breadcrumbs. Lay out on a pre-greased grill. Bake the fish in the oven at 350°F (180°C) for 20 minutes. Mix mayonnaise, horseradish, sugar, and salt to prepare the sauce.

SERVING

Lay out the lettuce leaves on a serving dish. Place the cooked fish on the lettuce and garnish it with corn. Decorate the dish with lemon slices and black olives. Serve the sauce separately in a gravy boat.

081 Portuguese Fish in a Cream Sauce

INGREDIENTS

17.5 OZ (500G) OF ANY SALTWATER FISH
3 TOMATOES
1 CARROT
1 CAN OF CRABMEAT
1 TBSP OF BUTTER
1 TBSP OF WHEAT FLOUR
5 FL OZ (150 ML) OF FISH BROTH OR MILK
SALT & GROUND BLACK PEPPER
PARSLEY, TARRAGON, & DILL
3 TBSP OF ANY KIND OF GRATED CHEESE
LETTUCE LEAVES & TOAST SLICES FOR SERVING

PREPARATION

Slice the fish and season with salt to taste. Cut the tomatoes into chunks and the carrots into thin slices.

Lay out the fish slices, alternating with tomatoes and carrots in a ring with crabmeat in the middle. Bake at 350°F (180°C) for 20 minutes. Melt butter in a pan. Stir in the flour and simmer for a few minutes. Add fish broth or milk. Season with salt and pepper and boil for a few minutes. Add chopped potherbs. Cover the fish and vegetables with mixture. Sprinkle with grated cheese and bake for 10 minutes.

SERVING

Place a lettuce leaf on a large plate and place the fish and vegetable ring on top. Serve with half slices of toast.

082 Fish Ring

INGREDIENTS

14 OZ (400G) OF ANY SALTWATER FISH FILLETS
SEA SALT & BLACK PEPPER
7 FL OZ (200 ML) OF VEGETABLE OIL
2 EGGS
POTHERBS FOR SERVING

BATTER:
SALT
4 FL OZ (125 ML) OF MILK
3.5 OZ (100G) OF FLOUR
4 EGGS

PREPARATION

Cut the fish fillets into small pieces and season them with salt and pepper. Roll the fish in flour and lightly fry it in oil. To prepare the batter, salt the milk, then add flour and the yolks of 4 eggs. Knead the dough. Whip the whites separately until stable foam appears and fold them gently into the batter. Dip the fish slices into this batter and fry them for 2 minutes on each side.

SERVING

Put the fish pieces in a ring on 2 individual pans. Break an egg in the middle of each pan. Bake it in the oven for 5-7 minutes. Serve the dish in the frying pan and decorate with potherbs.

083 Tuna Mousse in Apricot Halves

INGREDIENTS

6 CANNED APRICOT HALVES
1 CAN OF TUNA
5.5 OZ (150G) OF COTTAGE CHEESE
1 SMALL PURPLE ONION
A HANDFUL OF WALNUTS
6 CAPERS

PREPARATION

Strain the juice from the canned apricots. Mix the tuna and cheese in a blender. Add the onion and chopped walnuts. Fill the apricot halves with this mousse.

SERVING

Lay out the apricot halves in a row on 2 dessert plates. Fill them with mousse and place 2-3 capers on top.

084 Sea Bass Under Orange-Ginger Juice

INGREDIENTS

1 BUNCH OF SPINACH
3.5 OZ (100G) OF ASPARAGUS
1 TBSP OF BUTTER
1 TBSP OF OLIVE OIL
1 CLOVE OF GARLIC
½ TSP OF THYME
2 SEA BASS FILLETS
SALT & PEPPER
3 TBSP OF GINGER ROOT
7 FL OZ (200 ML) OF FRESH ORANGE JUICE
2 ORANGE RINGS WITH ZEST FOR SERVING
2 SPRIGS OF THYME

PREPARATION

Wash the spinach and remove any coarse stems. Wash the asparagus and peel it. Melt the butter and slightly fry the spinach leaves and asparagus. Roast the garlic and thyme in a pan. Add the fillets. Fry the fish on each side for 2 minutes. Season it with salt and pepper.

Grate the ginger root and squeeze the juice out. Mix with orange juice and simmer for 5 minutes.

SERVING

Put the spinach on 2 serving plates. Place the sea bass fillet and orange sprigs atop the spinach Add a sprig of thyme and asparagus. Pour over with orange and ginger juice.

085 Jack Krakowski Hake

INGREDIENTS

8 SMALL HAKE FISH
SALT & BLACK OR LEMON PEPPER
1 LEMON
8 SPRIGS OF DILL
2 MEDIUM TOMATOES
10 FL OZ (300 ML) OF SOUR CREAM
2 CLOVES OF GARLIC
4 OZ (120G) OF HARD CHEESE (CONTAINING AT
LEAST 45% FAT)
1 TBSP OF CHOPPED DILL
BREAD CRUMBS

PREPARATION

Wash the hake and remove the backbone. Season with salt and pepper and sprinkle with lemon juice. Put parchment paper on a baking sheet and grease with corn oil. Lay out the hake and put 2 sprigs of dill on each fish. Pour boiling water over tomatoes. Peel and chop them, then add half the sour cream, half the crushed garlic, and 1 oz (30g) of grated hard cheese. Rub 4 of the fish with this. Rub the other 4 fish with the same mixture, but replacing the tomatoes with chopped dill. Mix the remaining cheese with breadcrumbs and sprinkle all fish. Bake at 400°F (200°C) for 30 minutes.

SERVING

Arrange the baked hake on 2 platters, one with the tomato mixture and the other with sour cream and herbs. Decorate the dish with a lemon slice and a sprig of parsley.

086 Basic Hollandaise Sauce

INGREDIENTS

6 EGG YOLKS
10 OZ (300G) OF BUTTER
¼ CUP OF WATER
4 TBSP OF LEMON JUICE
SALT

PREPARATION

Pour the egg yolks into a thick saucepan. Add sliced butter and water. Simmer everything on low heat, stirring constantly, until the mixture has a liquid cream consistency. Add lemon juice and salt to your taste.

SERVE WITH

This sauce is served not only with fish and seafood, but also with cauliflower, asparagus, and artichokes.

087 Hollandaise with Citrus Juice

INGREDIENTS

2 FL OZ (50 ML) OF TANGERINE OR ORANGE JUICE
2 CUPS OF HOLLANDAISE SAUCE
ZEST
1 TSP OF BEET JUICE

PREPARATION

Add tangerine or orange juice to the hollandaise sauce, followed by zest and few drops of beet juice for color.

SERVE WITH

This sauce is served with fish and vegetable dishes.

088 Basic Fish Sauce

INGREDIENTS

2 CUPS OF FISH BROTH
1.5 OZ (40G) OF BUTTER
2 OZ (50G) OF FLOUR
½ ONION
½ CELERY STALK OR PARSLEY ROOT
2-3 WHOLE BAY LEAVES
4 WHOLE PEPPERCORNS
SALT

PREPARATION

Prepare saturated fish broth from fish fins, heads, bones, and skin. Melt 1 tablespoon of butter in a frying pan. Add flour and fry until it develops a nutty flavor. Gradually add the hot broth to the pan and stir constantly. Fry the onions and the roots mixed with flour-broth sauté. Add the spices and simmer everything for 50 minutes. Season with salt. Strain the sauce through a sieve and bring it back to a boil before letting it cool.

Keep the sauce in a glass container. It can be stored it in the refrigerator for 2-3 days. Use as needed.

089 Mushroom Fish Sauce

INGREDIENTS

3.5 OZ (100G) OF FRESH MUSHROOMS
2 WHOLE BAY LEAVES
3-4 WHOLE PEPPERCORNS
2 CUPS OF BASIC WHITE FISH SAUCE
1 ONION
2 TBSP OF DRY WHITE WINE
1 TBSP OF BUTTER
CHOPPED PARSLEY

PREPARATION

Boil mushrooms with bay leaves and pepper. Strain the broth through a sieve and add it to the fish sauce. Fry the onions and boiled mushrooms, and then add them as well. Simmer everything for 30 minutes. Strain the sauce through a sieve and return it to the pan. Add the wine and bring it to a boil. Add butter and chopped parsley, then let it cool.

SERVE WITH

This sauce goes well with boiled shrimp and hot fish dishes.

090 Provencal Sauce

INGREDIENTS

1 ONION
3.5 OZ (100G) OF FRESH MUSHROOMS
1 TBSP OF OLIVE OIL
2 CUPS OF BASIC FISH SAUCE
1 TBSP OF TOMATO PASTE
2 CLOVES OF GARLIC
1 TBSP OF BUTTER

PREPARATION

Fry the onion and chopped, boiled mushrooms in vegetable or olive oil for 5 minutes. Add fish sauce and tomato paste, and cook for 15 minutes. Add crushed garlic and butter when finished.

SERVE WITH

Provencal sauce is perfect for hot fish dishes.

Section III: Seafood

With aphrodisiacs, many kinds of seafood are recognized by the general public for their sexual properties. Most people think of oysters first, followed by shrimp, mussels, scallops, caviar, squid, and laminaria (kelp).

OYSTERS

Oysters contain a great deal of zinc and iron. Iron helps to transport oxygen throughout the blood vessels, while zinc stimulates metabolism and increases testosterone. These two elements affect both male and female libido very strongly. It is from this high concentration of zinc (16mg per 100g) that oysters have earned their reputation for being the king of seafood aphrodisiacs. Additionally, thanks to their combination of amino acids, bivalve mollusks can significantly improve male sexual health. It is reported that Casanova ate 50 oysters for breakfast daily.

Oysters caught in spring are considered to be the most potent. During this time, the shellfish is actively procreating, and its concentration of amino acids is at its highest.

SHRIMP

Nutrients in shrimp regulate blood circulation and support hormonal balance in men. Besides vitamins A, B1, B2, B3, B9, B12, C, D, and E, the list of trace minerals found in shrimp is almost endless and includes zinc, manganese, chromium, molybdenum, cobalt, nickel, fluoride, calcium, sodium, phosphorus, and sulfur.

Iodine content in these crustaceans is 100 times more concentrated than beef. Just 100g of shrimp contains a person's entire daily requirement of iodine and more than twice that of potassium. Taurine, which is found in energy drinks, is extracted from shrimp. Farm-raised shrimp have fewer useful nutrients because they are grown in captivity and given antibiotics.

MUSSELS

Mussels contain a high number of amino acids, particularly a type called mytilus. Mussels even contain the amino acid, D-aspartic, which is involved in releasing testosterone in men and progesterone in women. Some even say the amino acid profile in mussels is superior to any other food on earth. Additionally, mussels have a large amount of N-methyl-D-aspartate, which increases resistance to extreme situations and has antidepressant qualities.

Mussels contain taurine and arginine which directly affect the quality of sex. Arginine is involved in nitric oxide production. Nitric oxide has a strong relaxing effect on blood vessels which helps stimulate blood flow in the body and the pelvic organs in particular. This is not only good for all our organs but also contributes to the duration of sex.

The beneficial effects of arginine on all metabolic processes in the body were proven in 1998. Three American scientists received a Nobel Prize for their research. Arginine can be produced in the body, but only under ideal conditions. After age 50, the production of arginine diminishes.

SCALLOPS

In the Middle Ages, scallop shells were sold to pilgrims visiting the tomb of St. Jacob in the Spanish town of Santiago de Compostela. They were believed to attract good luck and bring good health. Vertically divided clamshells are also considered a symbol of femininity.

The most valuable parts of the scallops are the mantle and the adductor muscle. They are a valuable source of the natural minerals and trace elements iodine, iron, phosphorus, copper, zinc, manganese, cobalt, and calcium. Furthermore, scallops contain a whole multivitamin complex, as well as omega-3 and omega-6 polyunsaturated fatty acids. Scientists have proven that regular consumption of scallops by men helps to restore and maintain sexual function at a high level for a long time.

If you order scallops in a restaurant, tradition dictates that the waiter serves the dish to the man first, then to his companion. In Asian countries, scallops are valued for their ability to increase male potency. If you include scallop dishes in your diet regularly, this effect will last a long time!

FISH CAVIAR

Fish eggs or caviar contain a unique set of biologically active elements intended for the development of a new life. Of the total nutrients in caviar, 32% consists of a protein that is required for sperm production. Besides this protein, caviar contains vitamins A, D, and E, polyunsaturated fatty acids, folic acid, iodine, calcium, and phosphorus. Iodine and calcium promote serotonin production. So, thanks to its chemical composition caviar is capable of significantly improving the quality of sex.

Avoid overuse of caviar and be aware of preservatives used to increase shelf life. Always carefully read the label and do not buy caviar where the banned substance methenamine (E239) has been used as a preservative.

SQUID

According to ancient Greek mythology, there was an ordinary girl who seduced the sun god Apollo by giving him a dish prepared from squid. When the golden-haired god tasted it he became inflamed with passion for the girl. She had not realized the squid was a powerful aphrodisiac.

Squids are decapod cephalopods, the largest inverte- brates in the world. Their meat is much healthier than any other, including beef and chicken. Squid contains no fat or cholesterol, and its taurine content actually assists in reduc- ing cholesterol. Its meat is rich with phosphorus (250mg per 100g) which benefits the entire reproductive system.

Squid contains vitamins B1, B2, B4, B6, B9, C, and E, as well as trace elements such as zinc, iron, and iodine. Addi- tionally, squid helps build muscle mass and is invaluable for bodybuilders, because it has 18g of protein per 100g of meat. Squid dishes can be extremely tasty and unique.

A word of caution... Squid is not recommended people who are allergic to iodine, as it can cause severe reactions.

LAMINARIA (KELP)

Kelp is a powerful aphrodisiac thanks to its large con- centration of digestible iodine. This trace element plays an important role in the production of thyroid hormones. The thyroid is responsible for serotonin and hormones related to sexual health. Kelp is also rich in zinc, bromine, iron, magnesium, manganese, potassium, sulfur, and nitrogen, as well as folic, alginic, and pantothenic acids. You'll even get loads of vitamins A, B1, B2, B12, C, D, and E.

To prepare, place dry kelp in clean water at room tem- perature and leave for two hours. Drain the water and rinse the kelp to wash away any slime or sand. Dried and ground kelp also makes for a great salt substitute.

117

091 Squid with Breadcrumbs Appetizer

INGREDIENTS

17.5 OZ (500G) OF SQUID
2 CUPS OF BREADCRUMBS
½ CUP OF GROUND WALNUTS
2 EGGS
2 TBSP OF VEGETABLE OIL
2 TBSP OF WATER
½ CUP OF FLOUR
A HANDFUL OF SESAME SEEDS

SAUCE:
3 SLICES OF LEMON
3 TBSP OF MAYONNAISE
2 TSP OF CHILI SAUCE

PREPARATION

Clean squid and cut into rings. Mix breadcrumbs with walnuts. Whip eggs with vegetable oil and water. Bread the squid rings first in flour, then in egg, and then in the mix of breadcrumbs and nuts. Fry the squid in vegetable oil.

To prepare the sauce: peel and finely chop 3 lemon slices. Mix the mayonnaise, chili sauce, and chopped lemon slices. Fry sesame seeds in a pan until lightly browned.

SERVING

Place fried squid rings on a platter and sprinkle with roasted sesame seeds. Place a gravy boat to the side.

092 High Spirits Squid Salad

INGREDIENTS

1 HEAD OF CHINESE CABBAGE
2 BELL PEPPERS (RED & YELLOW)
3.5 OZ (100G) OF SQUID FILLETS
3.5 OZ (100G) OF KALE
2.5 OZ (75G) OF CANNED CORN
2 TBSP OF OLIVE OIL
JUICE OF ½ LEMON
SALT & PEPPER
A HANDFUL OF CRANBERRIES (OR ANY OTHER RED BERRIES) FOR SERVING

PREPARATION

Cut the leaves of the Chinese cabbage into squares approx. 1.5" (4cm) long. Slice the bell pepper into rings. Boil the squid fillets in salted water for 4-5 minutes. Cool them down and cut them into strips. Coarsely chop the kale. Add corn. Mix everything and dress with olive oil and lemon juice. Season the salad with salt and pepper.

SERVING

Put a leaf of Chinese cabbage into a dish and lay salad on top of it. Place a slice of lemon and a handful of cranberries beside the salad.

093 Colorful Squid Salad

INGREDIENTS

2 SQUIDS
2 FRESH CUCUMBERS
1 BUNCH OF LETTUCE
2 TOMATOES
3.5 OZ (100G) OF RED BEANS
SALT
POTHERBS

SAUCE:
2 FL OZ (50 ML) OF OLIVE OIL
JUICE OF ½ LEMON
1 TSP OF MUSTARD
1 TBSP OF SOY SAUCE
FINELY CHOPPED SPRING ONIONS.

PREPARATION

Boil the squids. Dip into cold water and peel them. Cut them into strips. Peel the cucumber into a spiral for decoration. To prepare the sauce: mix olive oil, lemon juice, mustard, and soy sauce in a blender. Add finely chopped spring onion.

SERVING

Lay out lettuce leaves around the perimeter and the bottom of a glass salad bowl. Place a layer of tomatoes sliced into squares, a layer of squid, a layer of cucumber, and a layer of beans. Season with sauce and decorate with chopped potherbs. Place 2 cucumber peel spirals around the salad bowl rim.

094 Green Spirit Squid Appetizer

INGREDIENTS

1 SQUID
SALT
1 CUCUMBER
¼ CUP OF CLEAR VINEGAR

PREPARATION

Boil the squid in salted water for 5 minutes. Strain through a sieve and rinse with cold water. Spirally peel the squid and cut it in half rings or strips.

To prepare green vinegar, grate the peeled cucumber and mix it with vinegar.

SERVING

Place the squid into a round platter. Pour green vinegar over the squid. Place a cucumber spiral beside it.

095 Squid on Nut Bed Appetizer

INGREDIENTS

2 SQUIDS
SALT
1 CUP OF CHOPPED WALNUTS
1 TSP OF OLIVE OIL
1 TSP OF SUGAR OR HONEY
DILL
2 LEMON SLICES
1 TSP OF CAPERS FOR SERVING

PREPARATION

Boil the squid in salted water for 3-5 minutes. Dip it in cold water and peel. Cut into thin strips. Crush the nuts in a blender or mortar. Mix thoroughly with olive oil and sugar or honey.

SERVING

Form round nut beds on 2 serving plates. Place the squids on top and sprinkle the dish with chopped dill. Place a slice of lemon and capers beside it.

096 Shrimp & Pumpkin Harmony Salad

INGREDIENTS

3.5 OZ (100G) OF COOKED PUMPKIN
3.5 OZ (100G) OF COOKED & PEELED SHRIMP
3.5 OZ (100G) OF SPINACH
2 RED OR ORANGE BELL PEPPERS
2 TBSP OF OLIVE OIL
JUICE OF 1 LEMON & A PINCH OF LEMON SALT
2 TSP OF SESAME SEEDS

LEMON SALT:
2 CLOVES OF GARLIC
1 LEMON
1 TBSP OF SEA SALT
2 OZ (50G) OF SWEET PEAS

PREPARATION

Coarsely grate the pumpkin. Mix with shrimp and chopped spinach. Slice the bell peppers into rings. Mix olive oil, lemon juice, and lemon salt to make a dressing.

To prepare lemon salt: crush the garlic and prepare the zest. Dry in the oven at 200°F (100°C) for 10 minutes. Crush the salt, sweet peas, zest, and garlic in a mortar or a blender.

SERVING

Place the pumpkin, shrimp, and spinach on a platter with bell pepper rings around. Pour over with sauce. Sprinkle with sesame seeds roasted in a frying pan for 2-3 minutes.

097 Sexy Shrimp Cocktail

INGREDIENTS

7-8 LARGE SHRIMP
SALT
1 TOMATO
1 GREEN OR YELLOW BELL PEPPER
½ AVOCADO
1 SMALL ONION
SEVERAL BASIL LEAVES

DRESSING:
BALSAMIC VINEGAR
OLIVE OIL

PREPARATION

Simmer peeled shrimp in salted water. Chop the tomato, pepper, and avocado into small cubes. Cut the onion into very thin half-rings. Tear the basil leaves with your hands and carefully mix all ingredients.

To prepare the dressing: mix the balsamic vinegar and olive oil.

SERVING

Put salad in a glass bowl. Dress with olive oil and vinegar.

098 Baltic Shrimp Salad

INGREDIENTS

7 OZ (200G) OF SHRIMP
SALT
7 TANGERINES
5 TBSP OF MAYONNAISE
1 APPLE
½ LEMON
3.5 OZ (100G) OF CELERY ROOT
LETTUCE LEAVES FOR SERVING

PREPARATION

Boil the shrimp in salted water and peel. To prepare the sauce: squeeze the juice from 3 peeled tangerines and mix with mayonnaise. Divide the remaining 4 tangerines into segments and remove the bitter white film. Peel the apple, and then slice and sprinkle it with lemon juice to avoid darkening. Finely chop the celery.

SERVING

Lay out the lettuce on the dish. Place the tangerine, apple, and cooked shrimp on top. Lay out the celery around the shrimp. Pour mayonnaise and tangerine juice sauce over everything. Adorn with lemon slices.

099 Shrimp in Sockets

INGREDIENTS

3.5 OZ (100G) OF BUTTER
17.5 OZ (500G) OF PEELED SHRIMP
3.5 FL OZ (100 ML) OF CREAM
BREADCRUMBS
A SPRIG OF DILL OR ANY OTHER POTHERB FOR SERV-
ING

PREPARATION

Grease porcelain or julienne dishes with butter. Put 2 tbsp of chopped shrimp into each dish. Cover with cream, sprinkle with breadcrumbs, and place a piece of butter on top. Bake in the oven at 350°F (180°C) for 7 minutes.

SERVING

Place everything on a flat dessert plate. Decorate with a sprig of dill or any other potherb.

100 Baked Shrimp in a Cream-Wine Sauce

INGREDIENTS

24.5 OZ (700G) OF SHRIMP
3 TBSP OF BUTTER
SALT & PEPPER
2 TBSP OF BRANDY
1 ONION
1 TBSP OF TOMATO PURÉE OR PASTE
1 WHOLE BAY LEAF
A PINCH OF SAVORY
5 FL OZ (150 ML) OF DRY WHITE WINE
3.5 FL OZ (100 ML) OF CREAM
A SPRIG OF DILL FOR SERVING

PREPARATION

Peel and rinse the shrimp. Fry in butter for 1 minute. Season with salt and pepper, and then pour brandy into the pan and flambé it. When the flame goes out, put finely chopped onion, tomato purée, bay leaf, and a pinch of savory. Pour wine over everything. Simmer on low heat for 5 minutes. Add the cream and simmer for another minute. Remove the shrimp from the pan and continue simmering the sauce for 1 more minute. Strain through a fine sieve.

SERVING

Put the shrimp on a preheated plate and pour the sauce over them. Decorate the dish with a sprig of dill.

101 Baked Mussels in Sour Cream Sauce

INGREDIENTS

24 FRESH MUSSELS
1 CARROT
1 SMALL PARSLEY ROOT
1 ONION
SALT
OIL FOR FRYING
2 OZ (50G) OF SOUR CREAM
2 OZ (50G) OF GRATED CHEESE
1 TBSP OF CHOPPED DILL OR PARSLEY
½ LEMON FOR SERVING

PREPARATION

Soak the mussels in cold water for 30 minutes, changing the water at least once. Add the carrot, parsley, and unpeeled onion to the water. Season with salt and boil for 12 minutes. Remove the mussel meat with a knife and fry in vegetable oil for 3 minutes. Add sour cream and stir. Put the mussels into baking molds and sprinkle with grated cheese. Bake at 350°F (180°C) for 15 minutes.

SERVING

Put the molds holding the mussels on dessert plates. Sprinkle with finely chopped dill or parsley. Place a fork and a dessert spoon on the side. Decorate the dish with a lemon quarter.

102 Clove Mussel Appetizer

INGREDIENTS

17.5 OZ (500G) OF COOKED & FROZEN MUSSELS
4 WHOLE CLOVES
2 CLOVES OF GARLIC
SALT
2 TBSP OF CHOPPED PARSLEY
2 OZ (50G) OF BUTTER
2 SPRIGS OF PARSLEY
SEVERAL OLIVES FOR SERVING

PREPARATION

Thaw the mussels and rinse them.

To prepare clove mixture: crush the cloves. Add crushed garlic, salt, and chopped parsley. Grease baking dishes with a small amount of butter. Melt the rest of the butter in a saucepan. Add the mussels to the baking dishes and sprinkle them with clove mixture. Pour butter over the mussels. Bake at 350°F (180°C) for 10-15 minutes.

SERVING

Place the baking dishes on a serving dish and decorate them with a sprig of parsley and olives.

103 Chicken Mussel Appetizer

INGREDIENTS

14 OZ (400G) OF COOKED & FROZEN MUSSELS
1 EGG
SALT & GROUND BLACK PEPPER
3.5 FL OZ (100 ML) OF MILK
1 TBSP OF BREADCRUMBS
1 TBSP OF FLOUR

TOMATO SAUCE:
1 ONION
PARSLEY
1 TBSP OF BUTTER
2 FL OZ (50 ML) OF DRY WHITE WINE
1 WHOLE BAY LEAF
1 CUP OF TOMATO SAUCE OR MILD KETCHUP

PREPARATION

Thaw and rinse the mussels. Add egg, salt, and pepper to milk and mix. Add mussels. Roll them in breadcrumbs and flour. Quickly fry in butter in a wok or saucepan.

To prepare the sauce: fry onion and parsley in butter for 2-3 minutes. Pour wine into the pan, and add the bay leaf, all-spice, and tomato sauce. Simmer the sauce for 10 minutes.

SERVING

Place the mussels on a platter. Place 2 saucers for each guest beside the dish. Serve the sauce on the side.

104 Crumb Mussels in Milk Sauce

INGREDIENTS

2-3 SHEETS OF FROZEN PUFF PASTRY
1 CUP OF MILK SAUCE
7 OZ (200G) OF MUSSELS
SALT & GROUND RED PEPPER
2 TBSP OF MELTED BUTTER
10 TSP OF CRACKERS
½ CUP OF CHOPPED POTHERBS

MILK SAUCE:
2 TBSP OF FLOUR
2 TBSP OF BUTTER
1.5 CUPS OF MILK

PREPARATION

Defrost the dough at room temperature. Cut circles for muffin tins with a larger diameter than the molds themselves. Bake the baskets at 350°F (180°C) for 10 minutes.

To prepare the milk sauce: fry flour in butter. Add hot milk. Simmer for 5 minutes while stirring. Add salt. Whip in a blender to remove lumps. Pour sauce over mussels and add red pepper. Lay out in baskets. Cover with melted butter and breadcrumbs. Bake at 350°F (180°C) for 5 minutes.

SERVING

Sprinkle serving dish with chopped potherbs. Place hot breadcrumb baskets on top.

131

105 Catalonian Mussels

INGREDIENTS

3 CLOVES OF GARLIC
2 FL OZ (50 ML) OF VEGETABLE OIL
14 OZ (400G) OF FROZEN MUSSELS
1 WHOLE BAY LEAF
SALT & BLACK PEPPER
2 TBSP OF COGNAC

SIDE DISH:
½ CUP OF BROWN RICE
1 TBSP OF VEGETABLE OIL

PREPARATION

Fry finely chopped garlic in a wok or deep frying pan for 3 minutes. Add boiled mussels, bay leaf, and pepper. Shortly before the mussels are cooked, season them with salt. Pour some cognac and flambé it.

Leave the brown rice to soak for 10 minutes. Drain the water and let the rice dry. Heat a tablespoon of vegetable oil in the saucepan. Fry the rice so that each paddy is covered with oil. Pour boiling water over everything and cook until the rice is tender. The rice should be crumbly and soft.

SERVING

Lay out the rice on 2 dishes with a culinary ring. Place the mussels around the ring and on top of the rice.

106 Scallop & Asparagus Salad

INGREDIENTS

3 MUSHROOM CAPS
3.5 OZ (100G) OF ASPARAGUS
7 OZ (200G) OF SCALLOPS
VEGETABLE OIL FOR FRYING
1.5 FL OZ (40 ML) OF DRY WHITE WINE
2 TBSP OF COTTAGE CHEESE
2 TSP OF SUGAR
1 OZ (25G) OF RED CAVIAR FOR SERVING

PREPARATION

Boil the mushroom caps and asparagus. Cut the scallops into large cubes and fry them in sunflower oil for a few minutes.

To prepare the sauce: simmer the wine over low heat. Add cottage cheese and sugar. Reduce the mixture until it reaches a thick honey state.

SERVING

Lay out the scallops on a plate. Pour sauce over the mushroom caps and asparagus. Decorate the dish with red caviar.

107 Scallops on a Rice Bed

INGREDIENTS

3.5 OZ (100G) OF RICE
A PINCH OF TURMERIC OR CURRY (OPTIONAL)
14 OZ (400G) OF SCALLOPS
3.5 OZ (100G) OF BUTTER
3.5 OZ (100G) OF ONIONS
2 BELL PEPPERS
3.5 FL OZ (100 ML) OF KETCHUP OR TOMATO SAUCE
CHOPPED PARSLEY FOR SERVING

PREPARATION

Boil the rice and add turmeric or curry powder. Fry the scallops in half the butter until golden.

To prepare the sauce: fry finely chopped onion and pepper in the remaining oil. After 3 minutes, add tomato sauce or ketchup to the rice. Simmer for 2-3 minutes.

SERVING

Put boiled rice on a large platter. Lay out the scallops on top of it. Pour sauce over the rice and scallops. Sprinkle the dish with chopped potherbs.

108 Scallop Fries

INGREDIENTS

24.5 OZ (700G) OF SCALLOPS
1 CUP OF MILK
3.5 OZ (100G) OF FLOUR
SALT & ALLSPICE TO TASTE
VEGETABLE OIL FOR FRYING
BUTTER
2 TSP OF CHOPPED THYME
1 TBSP OF CHOPPED PARSLEY FOR SERVING

PREPARATION

Cut the scallops lengthwise, then in half. Rinse and put them in milk for 5 minutes. Remove the scallops and bread them in flour mixed with salt and pepper. Fry in vegetable oil to a light brown color.

To prepare thyme herb butter: heat butter with thyme. Strain through a sieve.

SERVING

Place the scallops on a platter. Sprinkle them with thyme herb butter and parsley.

109 Scallop Sashimi Carpaccio in Cheese

INGREDIENTS

3.5 OZ (100G) OF HARD CHEESE
10 OZ (300G) OF FROZEN SCALLOPS
3.5 OZ (100G) OF CHEESE SAUCE
SEVERAL CHIVES FOR SERVING

CHEESE SAUCE:
3 TBSP OF BUTTER
3 TBSP OF FLOUR
½ TSP OF MUSTARD
2 CUPS OF MILK
1 CUP OF GRATED CHEDDAR CHEESE
SALT & PEPPER

PREPARATION

To prepare the cheese chips, grate the hard cheese and form chips with it on parchment paper. Bake these at 350°F (180°C) for 5-6 minutes. Slice the scallops.

To prepare the cheese sauce: melt the butter in a saucepan. Add flour and mustard. Stir and gradually add milk until smooth. Simmer for 2-3 minutes until thick. Add grated cheese and remove from heat. Season with salt and pepper.

SERVING

Lay out the scallops on 2 rectangular platters. Sprinkle with cheese sauce and cover with cheese chips. Spread the spring onions or chives on top of the scallops.

110 Scallop Carpaccio with Vanilla Sauce

INGREDIENTS

1 VANILLA BEAN
5 TBSP OF OLIVE OIL
10 SCALLOPS
JUICE OF ½ LEMON
1 TBSP OF GRATED PARMESAN CHEESE
4 SPRING ONIONS OR CHIVES FOR SERVING

PREPARATION

To prepare the vanilla sauce, open the vanilla bean and re-move the seeds. Put olive oil and the vanilla pod in a pan with a lid. Leave it in a dark place for a day to infuse. Wash and dry the scallops. Put them in a freezer for 20 minutes. Cut into thin slices.

SERVING

Take 2 rectangular sushi plates and lay out 5 cooked scal-lops in a row on each. Pour the vanilla sauce and lemon juice over them. Sprinkle the dish with grated parmesan cheese. Criss-cross the spring onion atop the dish.

111 Red Caviar Shrimp Salad

INGREDIENTS

½ AVOCADO
1.5 OZ (40G) OF CHERRY TOMATOES
4 ROYAL SHRIMP
1 TBSP OF OLIVE OIL
JUICE OF ½ LEMON
2 OZ (50G) OF ARUGULA
1 TBSP OF RED CAVIAR

PREPARATION

Cut the avocado into thin strips and the cherry tomatoes in half. Fry the shrimp in olive oil. Mix olive oil with lemon juice.

SERVING

Place the arugula on dishes. Lay out the tomato halves and shrimp on top. Randomly spread out the caviar on a plate. Drizzle the dish with a mixture of olive oil and lemon juice.

112 Caviar & Salmon Salad

INGREDIENTS

10 YOUNG POTATOES
3.5 OZ (100G) OF SMOKED SALMON
4 HARDBOILED QUAIL EGGS
1 BUNCH OF LETTUCE FOR SERVING
SALT & PEPPER
1 OZ (30G) OF CAVIAR
1 TBSP OF OLIVE OIL

PREPARATION

Boil the potatoes and slice them. Slice the salmon and cut the boiled eggs in half.

SERVING

Lay the lettuce leaves on 2 dishes and place the potato slices on top. Season them with salt and pepper. Lay out the salmon slices and put the quail eggs on them. Spread out the caviar on the salmon. Lightly sprinkle the salad with olive oil.

113 Red Caviar Pancakes

INGREDIENTS

17.5 OZ (500G) OF FLOUR
5 EGGS
2 OZ (50G) OF SUGAR
2 TSP OF SALT
34 FL OZ (1 LITER) OF MILK
3.5 FL OZ (100 ML) OF SUNFLOWER OIL
LETTUCE LEAVES & A SPRIG OF DILL FOR SERVING

FILLING:
1 OZ (30G) OF SALMON FILLET
1 OZ (30G) OF RED CAVIAR

PREPARATION

Mix flour, eggs, sugar, and salt into the milk to form dough. Knead the dough and let sit for 10-15 minutes. Pour the sunflower oil into the dough, thoroughly stirring. Form into small pancakes about 4" (10cm) in diameter and fry on medium heat.

To prepare the filling: mix finely chopped salmon fillet with red caviar. Wrap the pancakes around the filling so that it is still visible. Cut the pancakes in half before serving.

SERVING

Place lettuce on a large platter. One by one, lay out the pancakes on top of lettuce leaves. Decorate with a sprig of dill.

114 Red Caviar Charm Appetizer

INGREDIENTS

3.5 OZ (100G) OF CREAM CHEESE
7 OZ (200G) OF SOUR CREAM
3.5 OZ (100G) OF LIGHTLY SALTED SALMON
1 ONION
BUTTER FOR FRYING
4 HARDBOILED EGGS
A BUNCH OF DILL
3.5 OZ (100G) OF MAYONNAISE
SALT
2 OZ (50G) OF RED CAVIAR
CAPERS & LETTUCE FOR SERVING

PREPARATION

Mix cream cheese with sour cream and chopped salmon. Chop the onion and fry it in butter until soft. Slice hardboiled eggs, adding chopped dill and mayonnaise. Stir everything and season with salt to your taste.

SERVING

Place culinary rings on 2 flat plates and fill them in the following order: Layer 1: salmon with soft cheese. Layer 2: fried onions. Layer 3: eggs and potherbs. Remove the rings. Decorate the salads with caviar and surround them with capers. Place a sprig of dill on the side. Lay out lettuce leaves beside the salads. Decorate with caviar.

115 Red & White Caviar Appetizer

INGREDIENTS

1 LARGE DAIKON ROOT
SALT
1 LEMON
½ TSP OF DRIED OREGANO FOR SERVING
2 OZ (50G) OF RED CAVIAR
SEVERAL LEAVES OF MINT OR BASIL

PREPARATION

Cut or peel the daikon into long thin slices. Place it in hot, salted water, lightly soured with lemon juice. Boil for 3 minutes and dry on a paper towel.

SERVING

Take 2 dishes and sprinkle them with dried oregano. Lay out the nest of boiled daikon in the center of each plate. Place a handful of red caviar on top. Decorate with a leaf of mint or basil.

116 Sea Gift Salad

INGREDIENTS

1 SQUID
SALT
1 BELL PEPPER
1 RED ONION
3.5 OZ (100G) OF KELP
3.5 OZ (100G) OF GRATED CARROT
1 BUNCH OF LETTUCE LEAVES
3.5 OZ (100G) OF COOKED PEELED SHRIMP
2 SPRIGS OF PARSLEY OR CELERY FOR SERVING

SAUCE:
3 TBSP OF OLIVE OIL
1 TBSP OF BALSAMIC VINEGAR
SEA SALT & PEPPER

PREPARATION

Boil the squid for 2 minutes in salted water. Peel and cut it into strips. Cut the bell peppers and red onion into strips as well.

To prepare the sauce: mix the olive oil, vinegar, salt, and pepper. Combine the kelp, squid, bell pepper, onion, and grated carrot, and cover with sauce.

SERVING

Cover 2 serving plates with lettuce leaves and place the salad on top. Put the shrimp on top of the salad. Decorate the dish with a sprig of potherbs.

117 Exotic Kelp & Avocado Salad

INGREDIENTS

1 AVOCADO
1 BUNCH OF DILL
1 CLOVE OF GARLIC
JUICE OF ½ LEMON
7 OZ (200G) OF KELP
6 TBSP OF COOKED RED OR BROWN RICE
SALT & PEPPER
4 HARDBOILED QUAIL EGGS

PREPARATION

Clean the avocado and crush its pulp. Finely chop the dill and garlic. Mix the avocado, garlic, dill, and lemon juice in a blender. Combine the kelp with avocado, dill, and garlic. Mix all the vegetables with rice. Season the salad with salt and pepper to your taste.

SERVING

Divide the mixture into 2 portions in cups and press down with a spoon. Flip the cups on 2 serving plates. Lay out the quail eggs and sprigs of dill around the dish.

118 Kelp Salmon Rose Salad

INGREDIENTS

1 ONION
1 CLOVE OF GARLIC
3 TBSP OF OLIVE OIL
1 CARROT
14 OZ (400G) OF COOKED KELP
7 OZ (200G) OF SALMON CUT INTO SLICES
3 TBSP OF SOY SAUCE
1 TBSP OF WINE VINEGAR
1 CHILI PEPPER (OPTIONAL)
6 SPRIGS OF MINT FOR SERVING

PREPARATION

Chop the onion and garlic and fry them in olive oil. Grate the carrot. Mix kelp, half the salmon slices, and grated carrot with roasted onion and garlic. To prepare the dressing, mix the oil used for frying with soy sauce and vinegar. Add finely chopped chili pepper if desired. Season the salad.

SERVING

Place the salad on dishes. Decorate with salmon slices, shaping them in the form of roses. Lay out sprigs of mint under the salmon roses like rose leaves.

119 Kani Salad

INGREDIENTS

3 FRESH CUCUMBERS
7 OZ (200G) OF KELP
1 CAN OF CRABMEAT
JAPANESE MAYONNAISE
1 CAN OF ANY VARIETY OF CAVIAR

PREPARATION

Cut the cucumbers into strips and put on a paper towel to dry. Mix the kelp, crabmeat, and cucumbers. Dress the mixture with Japanese mayonnaise. Do not salt the salad.

SERVING

Put the salad into a salad bowl and decorate with caviar on top.

120 Sunomono Salad

INGREDIENTS

7 OZ (200G) OF FROZEN MUSSELS
1 DAIKON ROOT
1 CUCUMBER
3.5 OZ (100G) OF BOILED OCTOPUS
7 OZ (200G) OF KELP
1 TSP OF SESAME SEEDS
SEVERAL LEAVES OF ARUGULA FOR SERVING

DRESSING:
2 TBSP OF SOY SAUCE
1 TSP OF SPICY VINEGAR
2 FL OZ (50 ML) OF DRY WHITE WINE
2 TBSP OF SESAME OIL

PREPARATION

Thaw the mussels. Cut the daikon, cucumber, and octopus into strips. Open the mussels and cut them in half. Mix everything and add the kelp.

To prepare the dressing, combine the soy sauce, spicy vinegar, wine, and sesame oil. Dress the salad with this mixture.

SERVING

Lay out the salad with a culinary ring on 2 serving plates. Sprinkle with sesame seeds. Top with several arugula leaves.

Section IV: Nuts

Nuts are well-known aphrodisiacs because they have a beneficial influence on spermatogenesis. The most potent nuts are pine nuts, walnuts, and coconuts.

PINE NUTS

Pine nuts contain fat, proteins, starch, sugars, and vitamins. Their composition also includes oleic, linoleic, and linolenic acids. This protein is rich in the amino acids arginine, lysine, methionine, and tryptophan. They have a high content of tocopherols. Pine nuts contain vitamins A, B, C, D, and E, essential fatty acids, and minerals such as potassium, calcium, magnesium, zinc, cobalt, copper, and phosphorus. Pine nuts contain 55-66% healthy, cholesterol-free fats, and give a huge amount of energy for better sex.

WALNUTS

Walnuts contain many proteins, essential fatty acids, vitamins A and E, and B1 and B2. These are responsible for overall energy and sexual attraction. They also include minerals such as potassium, calcium, iron, sodium, magnesium, phosphorus, and iodine.

COCONUTS

Fresh coconut is a good aphrodisiac. When choosing a coconut, make sure it doesn't have any mold. If you bring the nut close to your ear and shake it, you should hear liquid splashing inside. This is a sign of freshness. Coconut also contains a high amount of vitamin E, which normalizes hormonal balance and increases libido.

ALMONDS

Almonds contain a significant amount of arginine. Eating 30 grams of almonds each week can increase sexual activity. Almonds contain about 26.22mg of vitamin E per 100g. Without this essential vitamin, our ability to reproduce diminishes, and we become indifferent to sex. Almonds also contain a large amount of healthy fats that provide energy for a sexual marathon.

121 Peter Simon Salad with Pine Nuts

INGREDIENTS

3 TOMATOES
3 BELL PEPPERS
3.5 OZ (100G) OF FETA OR MOZZARELLA CHEESE
3.5 OZ (100G) OF GREEN & BLACK PITTED OLIVES
SALT
PARSLEY
CELERY
3.5 OZ (100G) OF PINE NUTS
1 CUCUMBER

DRESSING:
OLIVE OIL
JUICE OF ½ LEMON

PREPARATION

Cut the tomatoes into slices. Peel the pepper and cut it into strips. Dice the cheese. Cut the olives in half and put several aside for serving. Stir everything, mixing in olive oil and lemon juice for dressing. Season with salt to your taste.

SERVING

Lay out the salad on 2 flat plates. Sprinkle with chopped parsley, celery, and pine nuts. Cut the cucumber into slices and place around the salad, alternating with the olive halves.

122 Energizing Pork with Pine Nuts

INGREDIENTS

1 TBSP OF WHITE FLOUR
14 OZ (400G) OF LEAN PORK
OLIVE OIL FOR FRYING
1.5 OZ (40G) OF PINE NUTS
JUICE & ZEST OF 1 LEMON
2 TBSP OF LIQUID HONEY
PARSLEY
LETTUCE LEAVES FOR SERVING
A MIX OF PEPPER, CORIANDER, NUTMEG, THYME, &
MARJORAM.
LETTUCE LEAVES FOR SERVING

PREPARATION

Combine the flour and spices. Dice pork into 1" (2cm) cubes. Heat olive oil in a pan, adding pork and seasoning with this mixture. Fry for 3 minutes, stirring continuously. Remove the pork from heat. Fry the pine nuts in olive oil and leftover pork juice. Add half the lemon zest, lemon juice, honey, and chopped parsley to the pine nuts and fry for 1 minute. Add pork back to the pan and fry for 3-5 minutes.

SERVING

Serve on large round dishes. Lay out the lettuce in the middle of the plate, placing the pork and pine nuts on top. Add lemon zest on top.

123 Pistou Pâté

INGREDIENTS

7 OZ (200G) OF PINE NUTS
2 CLOVES OF GARLIC
5 FL OZ (150 ML) OF OLIVE OIL
2 OZ (50G) OF COTTAGE CHEESE
1 SLICE OF TOAST (CUT INTO 2 TRIANGLES)
SEVERAL BASIL LEAVES FOR SERVING

PREPARATION

Grind all the ingredients in a blender, adding a small amount of water if necessary.

SERVING

Place the pâté in a pastry ring on a plate, lightly pressing it down. Remove the ring and put the triangles of toast in the center of the plate. Adorn with several basil leaves.

124 Heady Mushrooms with Pine Nuts

INGREDIENTS

2 CLOVES OF GARLIC
1 TBSP OF VEGETABLE OIL
17.5 OZ (500G) OF MUSHROOMS
1 TSP OF SMOKED PAPRIKA
SALT
1 TBSP OF BUTTER
5 FL OZ (150 ML) OF DRY WHITE WINE
1.5 OZ (40G) OF PINE NUTS

DRESSING:
JUICE & ZEST OF 1 LEMON
A FEW SPRIGS OF OREGANO OR THYME

PREPARATION

Finely chop the garlic and mix with vegetable oil. Add chopped mushrooms, smoked paprika, and salt. Grease a baking pan with butter and add the seasoned mixture. Bake at 350°F (180°C) for 5 minutes. Pour white wine over everything and continue baking for 15 minutes. Fry the pine nuts in a greased pan and set aside for serving.

To prepare the dressing: mix the juice and zest of 1 lemon with chopped oregano or thyme.

SERVING

Serve on individual dishes. Season with dressing and sprinkle with fried pine nuts.

125 Passionate Foreplay Salad

INGREDIENTS

14 OZ (400G) OF BOILED CHICKEN FILLET
1 AVOCADO
LETTUCE LEAVES
1 TANGERINE
5 CHOPPED HARDBOILED QUAIL EGGS
1 TBSP OF WALNUTS
1 TBSP OF PINE NUTS
JUICE OF ½ LEMON

DRESSING:
OLIVE OIL TO TASTE
5 FL OZ (150 ML) OF ORANGE JUICE
SALT

PREPARATION

Dice the boiled chicken and cut the pulp of the avocado into thin slices. Tear the lettuce with your hands. Peel the tangerine and split it into segments.

To prepare the dressing: mix the olive oil and orange juice. Season lightly with salt.

SERVING

Lay out the lettuce on a large serving dish with the chicken on top. Gently mix in quail eggs and tangerine slices. Sprinkle with chopped walnuts and pine nuts. Season with dressing. Sprinkle the avocado slices with lemon juice and serve.

126 Crudités Appetizer in Nut Sauce

INGREDIENTS

1 CUCUMBER
2 RADISHES
3.5 OZ (100G) OF RAW PUMPKIN OR BOILED SWEET
POTATO
1 TOMATO
1 BELL PEPPER
A HANDFUL OF SESAME SEEDS
POTHERBS

WALNUT SAUCE:
2 OZ (50G) OF WALNUTS
2 OZ (50G) OF ALMONDS
2 OZ (50G) OF SUNFLOWER SEEDS
1 CLOVE OF GARLIC
½ ORANGE
½ TSP OF CORIANDER OR DILL
SALT & GROUND BLACK PEPPER
2" (5CM) OF GINGER ROOT

PREPARATION

Chop the cucumber, radish, and pumpkin into slices. Finely chop the tomatoes and bell peppers.

To prepare the sauce: leave the nuts and sunflower seeds to soak in cold water overnight, and then rinse them under running water. Add garlic, juice of ½ the orange, coriander or dill, salt, and pepper, and grind everything in a blender. Add finely chopped ginger to the mix.

SERVING

Serve the dish on a large round plate. Lay out the vegetables around the plate without mixing. Leave the center of the plate empty by putting a glass in the middle before you begin. Sprinkle sesame seeds and potherbs around the perimeter. Remove the glass in the center and replace it with a gravy boat filled with nut sauce. Sprinkle the sauce with sesame seeds. Mix the vegetables into the sauce and enjoy.

127 Hawaiian Cocktail Salad

INGREDIENTS

1 CHICKEN BREAST
2 OZ (50G) OF DRIED WALNUTS
LETTUCE LEAVES
1 CAN OF PINEAPPLE SLICES
MAYONNAISE
2 OZ (50G) OF ANY VARIETY OF HARD CHEESE

PREPARATION

Boil the chicken breast. Let it cool and cut into large pieces. Chop the walnuts and tear the lettuce with your hands, setting aside 2 leaves for serving. Mix everything together with mayonnaise.

SERVING

Serve the cocktail-salad in small glass salad bowls or wine glasses. At the bottom of the salad bowl, place a leaf of lettuce adorned with a portion of salad. Decorate the dish with grated cheese.

128 Vegan Spinach Salad

INGREDIENTS

1 LARGE BUNCH OF SPINACH
JUICE OF ½ LEMON
1 TSP OF SOY SAUCE
2 OZ (50G) OF PEELED & ROASTED WALNUTS
1 CLOVE OF GARLIC
GROUND BLACK PEPPER

PREPARATION

Scald the spinach with boiling water and rinse it with cold water. Let it dry.

To prepare the dressing: mix the lemon juice, soy sauce, walnuts, and chopped garlic.

SERVING

Place everything on a flat plate and grind black pepper over it. Season to your preference with the dressing.

129 Waldorf Salad

INGREDIENTS

1 SMALL CELERY ROOT
2 MEDIUM-SIZED GREEN APPLES
3.5 OZ (100G) OF LARGE RED GRAPES
3.5 OZ (100G) OF CHERRIES
GROUND BLACK PEPPER
A HANDFUL OF WALNUTS

DRESSING:
3.5 OZ (100G) OF SOUR CREAM
3.5 OZ (100G) OF MAYONNAISE
JUICE OF 1 LEMON
A PINCH OF SUGAR

PREPARATION

Peel and coarsely grate the celery. Peel the green apple and cut it into small cubes before sprinkling with lemon juice. Cut the grapes and cherries in half, removing the seeds. Lightly mix the celery, grapes, apples, and cherries. Mix mayonnaise, sour cream, lemon juice, and sugar to make the dressing.

SERVING

Place the salad in salad bowls. Season with the dressing and black pepper. Sprinkle the salad with coarsely chopped walnuts.

130 Caramel Goat Cheese Corn Salad

INGREDIENTS

4 TBSP OF SUGAR
3 TBSP OF WHITE WINE VINEGAR
SALT
1 BOILED BEET
1 TBSP OF LIQUID HONEY
3 TBSP OF BALSAMIC VINEGAR
4 OZ (115 ML) OF OLIVE OIL
1 TSP OF DIJON MUSTARD
2 OZ (50G) OF GOAT CHEESE
1 CUP OF COOKED CORN
A HANDFUL OF WALNUTS

PREPARATION

Simmer the sugar over low heat, stirring constantly until it becomes liquid caramel. Add vinegar and 2 tablespoons of water. Season with salt. Let simmer for a couple of minutes. Dice the beet into large cubes and add it to the caramel. Mix everything and continue simmering for another minute.
To prepare the dressing: whip the honey, balsamic vinegar, and 1 tablespoon of olive oil using a whisk. Add mustard to your taste. Drizzle with olive oil and serve with salt.

SERVING

Place the caramelized beet and goat cheese in a deep dish. Add the corn and drizzle it with honey dressing, gently mix everything. Sprinkle with coarsely chopped walnuts.

131 Fish Fondue with Coconut Banana Sauce

INGREDIENTS

1 OZ (30G) OF COCONUT MEAT OR FLAKES
1 HOT PEPPER OF ANY VARIETY
2 TBSP OF VEGETABLE OIL
1 BANANA
5 OZ (150G) OF SOUR CREAM
5 OZ (150G) OF MAYONNAISE
SALT & WHITE PEPPER
3.5 OZ (100G) OF FLOUR
2 EGGS
4 FL OZ (120 ML) OF BEER
14 OZ (400G) OF ANY SALTWATER FISH FILLET
14 OZ (400G) OF SHRIMP

PREPARATION

Fry coconut pulp flakes until golden. Finely chop hot pepper and fry in vegetable oil. Peel the banana and knead into a purée. Mix the purée with sour cream and mayonnaise. Add salt and pepper to your taste. Add coconut and pepper to the banana. In a mixer, combine flour, eggs, salt, and beer into the batter. Slice the fish into portions and dry with a paper towel. Sprinkle shrimp with lemon juice.

SERVING

Prepare 2 individual plates. Heat the oil in a fondue pan. Lay out the fish and shrimp on the plates. At the serving table, dip the fish or shrimp in the batter and fry them in oil. Serve the coconut banana sauce separately.

132 Fresh Flavor Coconut Salad

INGREDIENTS

FRESH MEAT OF ½ COCONUT
1 SMALL ONION
2 CUCUMBERS
SALT
½ TSP OF GROUND RED & BLACK PEPPER

PREPARATION

Smash the coconut meat into mush in a blender. Cut the onion and cucumbers into thin half-rings. Mix these together with the coconut pulp and lightly season with salt and pepper.

SERVING

Line the coconut shell halves with foil and fill them with salad.

133 No-Bake Canadian Nanaimo Dessert Bars

INGREDIENTS

FIRST LAYER:
3.5 OZ (100G) OF BUTTER
2 OZ (50G) OF SUGAR
5 TBSP OF COCOA
1 EGG
7 OZ (200G) OF SHORTBREAD
2 OZ (50G) OF WALNUTS
3 OZ (80G) OF GRATED COCONUT MEAT OR FLAKES

SECOND LAYER:
1 CUP OF MILK
3.5 OZ (100G) OF BUTTER
7 OZ (200G) OF POWDERED SUGAR
1 TBSP OF ORANGE ZEST FOR THE PUDDING
3 TBSP OF INSTANT VANILLA PUDDING MIX
ZEST OF 1 ORANGE FOR SERVING

THIRD LAYER:
3.5 OZ (100G) OF DARK CHOCOLATE
2 TBSP OF BUTTER

PREPARATION

First layer:

Melt the butter, sugar, and cocoa powder in a saucepan. Whip 1 egg with a whisk and pour it in a thin stream into the buttery mixture. Simmer the mixture until thick for 1 minute and then remove from heat. Grind the shortbread in a blender or with a rolling pin, and then stir it into the buttery mixture. Add chopped walnuts and grated coconut or coconut flakes. Line a deep baking pan with foil or cling film. Pour the coconut mixture to form the first layer, tamping it down by hand. Refrigerate the mix.

Second layer:

Prepare the instant pudding using the milk. Whip softened butter with sugar, gradually adding the cooled pudding and orange zest. Pour this mixture over the first layer in the baking pan. Refrigerate once more.

Third layer:

Melt the chocolate and butter. Pour the mixture over the first two layers in the baking pan. Refrigerate again for a couple of hours.

For serving, arrange orange zest into thin strips and boil in a sugar syrup. Leave it on a platter to cool.

SERVING

Use a culinary ring to cut 2 round portions. Place them on dessert plates. Decorate with strips of orange zest. You can also cut the dessert into rectangles and decorate with orange zest strips.

134 Bankokko Cakes

INGREDIENTS

3 OZ (80G) OF MELTED BUTTER
3 OZ (80G) OF SUGAR
1 EGG
7 OZ (200G) OF FLOUR
½ TSP OF BAKING POWDER
2 BANANAS
3 EGGS
8 OZ (240G) OF GRATED COCONUT MEAT OR FLAKES
POWDERED SUGAR
2 SPRIGS OF MINT FOR SERVING

PREPARATION

Mix the butter with half the sugar and 1 egg. Mix the flour and baking powder. Gradually add the dry ingredients to the buttery mixture, kneading into a soft dough. Press the dough into a shallow baking pan to approx. 2" (5cm) thick. Bake at 350°F (180°C) for 15 minutes. Peel the bananas and cut them into slices. Mix the remaining 3 eggs with the remaining sugar and coconut. Place the banana slices on the dough and cover everything with the coconut mixture. Smooth the surface with a knife and return it to the oven for 20 minutes.

SERVING

Cut the cake into individual portions. Sprinkle with powdered sugar and decorate with sprigs of mint.

135 Coconut Halawa

INGREDIENTS

1 LARGE COCONUT OR 7 OZ (200G) OF COCONUT
FLAKES
3.5 OZ (100G) OF BUTTER
17 FL OZ (500 ML) OF MILK
9 OZ (270G) OF SUGAR
1.5 OZ (40G) OF ANY NUTS FOR SERVING

PREPARATION

Split the coconut into 2 halves and smash its meat in a
blender. Melt the butter in a saucepan and add the coconut
meat. Fry the mixture for 10 minutes on low heat. Meanwhile, simmer milk and sugar over low heat to make syrup.
Pour the hot syrup into the buttery coconut mixture. Stir
and continue simmering for another 10 minutes. Let it cool.

SERVING

Line the coconut shell with foil and fill it with the mixture.
Decorate with roasted nuts.

136 Almond Fragrance Salad

INGREDIENTS

1 BUNCH OF SPINACH
7 OZ (200G) OF FRESH MUSHROOMS
7 OZ (200G) OF CHERRY TOMATOES
⅓ CUP OF ALMONDS
2 TBSP OF OLIVE OIL
½ TSP OF BALSAMIC VINEGAR
A PINCH OF SEA SALT
FRESHLY GROUND BLACK PEPPER
1 TBSP OF ALMOND FLAKES AS GARNISH

PREPARATION

Wash the spinach leaves under running water and tear them with your hands. Wash the mushrooms and cut them into slices. Wash and cut the cherry tomatoes in half.

To prepare the dressing: fry almonds and mix in a blender with olive oil, balsamic vinegar, sea salt, and pepper.

SERVING

Put the spinach in a large dish and top it with mushrooms and cherry tomatoes. Drizzle with dressing and sprinkle with almond flakes.

137 Sea Salad with Almond Petals

INGREDIENTS

2 SQUIDS
14 OZ (400G) OF CUTTLEFISH MEAT
SEA SALT & BLACK PEPPER
2 CLOVES OF GARLIC
3.5 FL OZ (100 ML) OF WHITE WINE
2 OZ (50G) OF ALMONDS
3 CUCUMBERS
3.5 OZ (100G) OF ARUGULA
5 FL OZ (150 ML) OF OLIVE OIL
LETTUCE LEAVES FOR SERVING

PREPARATION

Clean the squids. Cut the first into pieces 1" (2.5cm) long. Cut the other into rings. Slice the cuttlefish. Heat a frying pan and sprinkle it with dry sea salt. Put the seafood in and fry on low heat for 5 minutes. Season everything with pepper. Add finely chopped garlic and wine near the end of frying and wait for it to evaporate. Remove from the heat.

Lightly fry the almonds. Cut the cucumbers into circles. Mix the cucumbers, arugula, and seafood in a bowl. Season everything with olive oil.

SERVING

Put the mix in a large salad bowl over lettuce. Sprinkle it with almonds and decorate it with squid rings.

138 Cauliflower & Almond Salad

INGREDIENTS

1 HEAD OF CAULIFLOWER
3.5 FL OZ (100 ML) OF OLIVE OIL
SALT
⅓ TSP OF GROUND CINNAMON
⅓ TSP OF GROUND ALLSPICE
1 OZ (30G) OF ALMONDS
1 POMEGRANATE
1 CELERY STALK
1 ½ TSP OF MAPLE SYRUP
1 TBSP OF SHERRY VINEGAR
A FEW SPRIGS OF PARSLEY

PREPARATION

Cut the cauliflower into florets and cover with 3 tbsp of olive oil. Season with salt, cinnamon, and allspice. Bake in the oven at 350°F (180°C) for 30 minutes until golden. Fry the almonds and chop them. Remove the pomegranate seeds from the fruit. Cut the celery stalk into thin pieces. Prepare the dressing with olive oil, maple syrup, and sherry vinegar.

SERVING

Take 2 large flat dishes and put salad bowls on them. Divide the cauliflower in the salad bowls and sprinkle with pomegranate seeds. Season with dressing, and sprinkle in the almonds and celery.

139 Almond Bomb Salad

INGREDIENTS

1 ORANGE
½ CUP OF GREEN SEEDLESS GRAPES
1 CUP OF ALMONDS
1 BUNCH OF LETTUCE
2 BUNDLES OF SPINACH
½ CUP OF CHOPPED SPRING ONIONS

DRESSING:
5 FL OZ (150 ML) OF OLIVE OIL
1.5 FL OZ (40 ML) OF ORANGE JUICE
3 TBSP OF LEMON JUICE
3 TBSP OF LIQUID HONEY
1 TSP OF CELERY SEEDS
1 TSP OF DRY MUSTARD
SEVERAL SPRING ONIONS

PREPARATION

Peel the orange and cut it into slices. Cut the grapes in half. Fry the almonds and coarsely chop them. Cut the lettuce and spinach. Mix the spinach, orange slices, grapes, spring onions, almonds, and lettuce in a mixing bowl. Mix the olive oil, orange juice, lemon juice, honey, celery seed, and dry mustard in a large bowl. Combine all the ingredients.

SERVING

This salad looks best on a rectangular dish. Serve the salad over lettuce on a serving plate and sprinkle it with dressing. Decorate the top of the dish with spring onions.

140 Mango Parfait with Candied Almonds

INGREDIENTS

14 OZ (400G) OF CANNED MANGO
2 EGG YOLKS
3.5 OZ (100G) OF SUGAR
½ TSP OF VANILLA SUGAR
1 FL OZ (30 ML) OF WATER
7 FL OZ (200 ML) OF 33% FAT CREAM
2 OZ (50G) OF ALMONDS

PREPARATION

Blend the mango and strain through a sieve. Mix the yolks with half the sugar. Add vanilla sugar and half the mango purée. Whip mixture until frothy. Transfer to a pot, add water, and let simmer for 10 minutes, stirring constantly. Let cool. Whip cream until stable peaks appear. Combine with mango yolk mixture and freeze for 3 hours. Whip mango ice cream and freeze in silicone molds.

To prepare the candied almonds: dissolve remaining sugar in water and pour in a saucepan. Simmer until syrup reaches a golden color. Chop and fry almonds. Add to caramel and mix. Grease parchment and put the caramel-nut mixture on it. Smooth and let cool. Mix in a blender.

SERVING

Spread roasted nuts on dessert plates. Put mango ice cream on top. Decorate with any berries you have.

Section V: Fruits

PINEAPPLE

Pineapples contain the enzyme bromelain, which is great for digestion. Pineapples also contain B vitamins to help increase physical strength and energy, which are obviously important if prolonged lovemaking is the goal.

AVOCADO

Avocado, or the alligator pear, is a very strong aphrodisiac. In ancient times, it was used to increase potency and fertility, so it was excluded from the diet of Spanish colonizers. The ancient Aztecs called it "the testicle tree" because the fruit hangs in pairs like testicles.

The main substances contained in avocados are phytosterols which awaken sexual desire in both men and women. Avocados also contain large amounts of carotenoids, lutein, beta-carotene, glutathione, and zeaxanthin. These all have high antioxidant properties. It also contains vitamins A, B1, B2, B3, B6, C, D, and K, as well as trace elements of calcium, potassium, iron, magnesium, sodium, and phosphorus. 30% of an avocado is healthy plant fat, which adds more energy to any physical activity. Its glutathione content saturates the tissues and organs with oxygen.

QUINCE

All kinds of quince, especially the sweet ones, enhance the libido and increase sexual activity. You can easily cook fragrant jellies and marmalades with this wholesome fruit, which are as delicious as they are healthy.

The pulp of this fruit contains carotenoids, the source of vitamin A. It also contains flavonoids, potassium, iron, and large amounts of vitamin C (30mg per 100g). Quince is full of fragrant essential oils that give it a delicate nutty flavor. Medieval monks thought quince jam was a powerful aphrodisiac. Roman gourmet cooks stored quince in jars of honey and wine and then ate it as an aphrodisiac. Cook this fruit with meat for an excellent non-traditional dish.

WATERMELON

The juicy pulp of watermelon contains citrulline, which dilates blood vessels and stimulates blood circulation in a similar way to Viagra. Watermelon contains vitamins A, B1, B2, B3, B6, B9, C, and E. In addition, watermelon pulp contains iron salts, copper, phosphorus, potassium, zinc, and folic acid. It has the largest amount of folic acid among all foods and the second highest iron content after spinach.

Watermelon has the highest lycopene content of any food. This potent antioxidant helps treat male infertility.

BANANA

This fruit is not only an aphrodisiac but looks like one because of its phallic shape! Bananas include enzymes that strengthen the male libido and also vitamin B6, which treats female anorgasmia. Bananas directly affect libido because they contain the enzyme bromelain and high levels of potassium, which stimulate serotonin. Also, bananas give energy from fructose, glucose, and sucrose.

Drink a banana milkshake before a date. Put on an erotic show by peeling and eating a banana. Don't throw away the peel, as it contains bufotenine, which enhances libido. In ancient times, it was used for creating love potions.

GRAPES

Grapes contain a record amount of natural boron, which increases testosterone levels and improves endurance during extended sexual encounters. Pekmez is boiled grape juice, which is thickened like syrup but does not contain any added sugar. Pekmez contains a lot of chromium, which is involved in spermatogenesis. It improves sperm quality and quantity. In Turkey, carob pekmez is made from grapes and black mulberries.

To prepare pekmez at home, simply squeeze the juice from 5kg of fresh grapes. Put the juice in a saucepan and simmer for 15 minutes. Add 300g of white clay. Remove the saucepan from heat and leave it to infuse for 5 hours. Carefully drain the juice into another pan and boil until it resembles liquid honey. Remove foam. Let it cool and pour into jars. Pour pekmez over the grape skins, cover the jar with cheesecloth and place it in a cool place for 10 days. You will get a wonderful natural grape vinegar. To prepare carob pekmez, soak carob tree pods in grape juice and heat until syrupy.

POMEGRANATE

Pomegranates have been known since ancient times as aphrodisiacs. According to ancient mythology, the god of the underworld, Pluto, did not want to lose his beloved Proserpine, so he gave her pomegranates.

A study in 2007 proved that pomegranates and pomegranate juice could help men with erectile dysfunction due to the fact that it increases sperm production and improves erection quality. Doctors recommend drinking pomegranate juice or eating pomegranates for 4 weeks, taking a 2-week break, and consuming it for another 4 weeks. Scientists have also discovered several active ingredients which are similar to female sex hormones and assist with sexual arousal.

DURIAN

Durian is a fruit from Southeast Asia, which is famous for having a heavenly taste but an awful smell. Some gourmets have likened its fragrance to that of a spicy cheese. This exotic fruit is recognized as the most powerful aphrodisiac among all the fruits in the world, and it works for both men and women.

In Malaysia, there is a saying that when a durian falls from a tree, sarongs fly up! It is claimed that its effects are felt within just 1 or 2 hours. Durian tastes like a caramel cream dessert, but has many more vitamins and minerals than the alternative. Be warned though: don't eat durian every day unless you want to find yourself in a constant state of sexual desire!

FIGS

Figs contain flavonoids, polyphenols, and antioxidants that can prolong pleasure during sexual intercourse. They also have magnesium, potassium, zinc, and vitamin E, which are very important for sexual health for both men and women alike. The shape of the fruit even resembles male testicles. Fig seeds contain substances which strengthen sexual endurance, so you and your lover can enjoy each other's embrace all night if you like.

STRAWBERRY

Strawberries soaked in champagne are a cliché of any romantic evening. However, there is a good reason for it.

Carbon dioxide in champagne combined with sugar from the strawberries increases production of female hormones, and thus, sexual desire.

Strawberry seeds contain zinc, which is involved in testosterone production and spermatogenesis. The endorphins contained in strawberries sharpen the senses. Wild strawberries with white port wine are a classic combination for any romantic dinner. Bright, red strawberries look sexy, and are used as a sexual symbol in popular media.

KUMQUAT

To experience the full flavor of this delicious fruit, eat it with the skin on. The juicy flesh of a kumquat has a sour taste, while its skin is sweet. You will experience the full range of sensations with each bite because it is saturated with essential oils. Kumquat is the smallest citrus fruit. It contains zinc, calcium, copper, pectin, vitamin C, and flavonoids. Kumquat has a positive effect on the nervous system, creating a positive mood and high spirits. Another bonus with this exotic fruit is it eliminates hangovers. The Japanese kumquat, Maeve, is the most powerful of all.

LYCHEE

Lychee has a long-standing positive reputation in China and other parts of the East. Lychees contain copper, potassium, phosphorus, iron, sulfur, iodine, fluorine, nicotinic acid, and vitamins C, B1, and B2. The rough peel is easily removed, making for a convenient and fun snack any time of day. Lychee are called the fruit of love in many Eastern countries for good reason.

MANGO

According to Asian legend, the god Shiva cultivated the mango tree and gave it to his beloved. People in India and Pakistan believe Eve tempted Adam with a mango. For 4,000 years, mangos were considered one of the most powerful aphrodisiacs. In modern India, it is recommended that men who have sexual problems consume this fruit often.

RASPBERRIES

Raspberries contains a lot of vitamin C, as well as B3, B9, and E. Besides zinc, raspberries are rich in potassium, phosphorus, magnesium, chlorine, selenium, copper, and calcium. They also contain the antioxidant anthocyanin, which strengthens the capillaries and blood flow to the sexual organs. Raspberries neutralize the destructive effects of free radicals which destroy cellular structure. Raspberries also help to get rid of the symptoms of a hangover, as they contain fruit acids such as malic and citric.

Raspberries are important for women because they normalize the uterus muscles. This is especially important if you are trying to get pregnant. Raspberries are a wonderful source of folic acid, which is important during the early stages of pregnancy because it helps the fetus to develop properly.

You can use raspberries to prepare smoothies, soft drinks, fruit salads with yogurt and honey, buttermilk, or just juice. Adding a little ice and a sprig of mint or lemon balm will add flavor to this versatile berry, making it a favorite treat wherever it is available.

DATES

The fruits of the date palm were considered a source of sexual power in ancient times. That's all thanks to their energy reserve of carbohydrates, which makes up 50 to 70% of the whole weight of the fruit. Dates are the sweetest fruit on Earth. According to the story One Thousand and One Nights, dates can give strength even to the most decrepit old men.

Dates contain vitamins A, B1, B2, and C, as well as folic acid, phenolic compounds, and the trace elements zinc, manganese, copper, selenium, and iron. Dates are recommended for couples wishing to have children because they improve sperm count and duration of sex, but you don't need to be trying to conceive in order to reap their enjoyment-enhancing benefits.

BILBERRY

Bilberries contain polyphenols which do a great job of relaxing blood vessels and improving circulation throughout the body. Normal blood flow is, of course, essential for quality erections. For maximum potency, it is recommended that you eat a portion of bilberries at least 3-4 times a week.

141 Atlantis Salad

INGREDIENTS

1 ONION
1 TBSP OF VINEGAR
SALT
SUGAR
2 EGGS
½ CUP OF MILK
9 OZ (250G) OF FLOUR
17.5 OZ (500G) OF ANY VARIETY OF CRABMEAT
OLIVE OIL FOR FRYING
½ SMALL PINEAPPLE
6 CHERRY TOMATOES
3.5 OZ (100G) OF OLIVES
1 BUNCH OF LETTUCE
1 TSP OF SESAME SEEDS FOR SERVING
LEMON SLICES FOR SERVING

DRESSING:
½ CUP OF OLIVE OIL
1 TBSP OF MUSTARD
1 TSP OF BALSAMIC VINEGAR
1 TSP OF LEMON JUICE
1 TSP OF SESAME OIL
1 CHILI PEPPER (OPTIONAL)

PREPARATION

Cut the onion into thin rings. Mix vinegar with ½ tsp of salt and ½ tsp of sugar. Marinate the onions in this mixture for 25 minutes. Prepare batter from the eggs, milk, and flour. Beat these ingredients with a mixer. Dip the crabmeat in the batter and fry it in olive oil until crisp. Peel the pineapple and cut it into small cubes. Cut the cherry tomatoes in half and the olives into rings. Cut the crabmeat into small pieces.

To prepare the dressing, mix olive oil, mustard, balsamic vinegar, lemon juice, and ½ teaspoon of sesame oil. Optionally, remove the seeds from the chili pepper and finely chop it. Add it to your taste.

SERVING

Lay out the lettuce on a large platter. Put the pineapple, pickled onion, crabmeat, cherry tomatoes, and olives on top. Drizzle the salad with dressing and sprinkle it with sesame seeds. Decorate the dish with lemon slices.

142 Tropical Memories Dessert

INGREDIENTS

1 BANANA
1 SMALL PINEAPPLE
1 TBSP OF BUTTER
1 TBSP OF HONEY
POWDERED SUGAR & COCOA POWDER
7 OZ (200G) OF ICE CREAM
2 TBSP OF FRUIT OR BERRY SYRUP
ANY FRUIT (LEMON, ORANGE, KIWI, ETC.) FOR DEC-
ORATION.

PREPARATION

Peel both the banana and pineapple, and cut them into thick rings. Melt the butter in the saucepan with honey. Fry the pineapple rings in this mixture on both sides.

SERVING

Prepare 2 plates. Sprinkle half of each plate with powdered sugar. Sprinkle the other half with cocoa powder. Lay out pineapple rings on top. Put a scoop of ice cream on the pineapple and pour fruit or berry syrup over it. Stick a skewer in the pineapple. You can also put any fruit such lemon or orange rings, or slices of kiwi or strawberries to the side.

143 Food of the Gods Cocktail Salad

INGREDIENTS

½ SMALL PINEAPPLE
2 BANANAS
4 KIWIS
2 TBSP OF ANY VARIETY OF CRUSHED NUTS
2 TBSP OF POWDERED SUGAR
2 TSP OF VANILLA SUGAR
2 SPRIGS OF MINT FOR SERVING
LEMON JUICE & A SPRIG OF MINT FOR SERVING

DRESSING:
ANY FRUIT SYRUP
LEMON JUICE TO TASTE

PREPARATION

Peel the pineapple. Cut all the fruit into cubes. Mix the nuts, powdered sugar, and vanilla sugar.

SERVING

Place the glasses upside down. Dip them in lemon juice, then in sugar. Fill the glass with the fruit salad. Pour your favorite fruit syrup and lemon juice over it. Decorate the dish with a sprig of mint.

144 Pineapple Chia Smoothie

INGREDIENTS

1 PINEAPPLE
1 BANANA
1 ½ CUPS OF FRUIT YOGURT
1 TSP OF CHIA SEEDS
A FEW SPRIGS OF MINT FOR SERVING

PREPARATION

Peel the pineapple and cut it into cubes. Peel the banana and cut it into thick rings. Put 1 cup of fruit yogurt in a blender bowl. Add pineapple, banana, the remaining yogurt, and chia seeds to the bowl. Beat all the ingredients into a foam.

SERVING

Pour the smoothie into cappuccino glasses and decorate with mint leaves.

145 Pineapple Tiramisu in Coconut Boats

INGREDIENTS

1 FRESH PINEAPPLE
2 EGGS
2 OZ (50G) OF SUGAR
5 OZ (150G) OF MASCARPONE
5 OZ (150G) OF LADYFINGERS
3.5 FL OZ (100 ML) OF COCONUT LIQUEUR
1 SMALL COCONUT
COCOA FOR SERVING

PREPARATION

Peel the pineapple and cut it into cubes. Separate the egg yolks from their whites. Beat the yolks with sugar. Gradually add mascarpone to the yolks. Whip the whites and fold them into the yolk mix. Soak the biscuits in coconut liqueur. Split the coconut in half. Remove the meat and chop it into small pieces.

SERVING

Put a small amount of cream on the bottom of the coconut shells. Layer the ingredients in the following order on top of the cream: ladyfingers, pineapple, ladyfingers, pineapple, and cream. Sprinkle the last cream layer with cocoa and decorate with pieces of coconut meat. Refrigerate for 5 hours.

146 Jamantinos Avocado Salad

INGREDIENTS

1 AVOCADO
1 TBSP OF LEMON JUICE
1 CUCUMBER
1 TOMATO
1 YELLOW BELL PEPPER
3.5 OZ (100G) OF SHRIMP
2 OZ (50G) OF SALMON FILLET
3.5 OZ (100G) OF BLUE CHEESE
SALT & PEPPER
1 TBSP OF OLIVE OIL
1 TSP OF WINE OR BALSAMIC VINEGAR
2 HARDBOILED QUAIL EGGS

PREPARATION

Cut the avocado in half. Remove pit and pulp. Cut the pulp into cubes and sprinkle with lemon juice. Cut the cucumber and tomato into cubes. Slice the bell pepper into strips. Boil the shrimp. Peel and cut them into pieces. Cut the salmon into cubes. Cut the cheese into triangles. Mix avocado with vegetables, shrimp, and salmon. Add salt and pepper.

To prepare the dressing: mix oil, vinegar, salt, and pepper.

SERVING

Lay out lettuce leaves on 2 dishes. Place the salad on top and pour dressing over. Place slices of blue cheese and quail eggs on the side. Pour the sauce in drops around the salad.

147 Avocado Salad with Poppy Seeds

INGREDIENTS

1 TSP OF POPPY SEEDS
1 AVOCADO
7 OZ (200G) OF FRESH STRAWBERRIES
2 FRESH CUCUMBERS
JUICE OF 1 LEMON OR LIME
1.5 OZ (40G) OF OLIVE OIL
1.5 FL OZ (40 ML) OF WALNUT OIL
PEPPER

PREPARATION

Rinse the poppy seeds and pour boiling water over them. Set aside for 20 minutes. Remove the avocado pulp and sprinkle it with ½ the lemon or lime juice. Slice the avocado, strawberries, and cucumber.

Prepare the dressing by mixing lemon juice, olive oil, walnut oil, and pepper. Strain the water from the poppy seeds. Add poppy seeds to the dressing and stir it thoroughly.

SERVING

Place the avocado in a salad bowl. Lay out a semicircle of strawberries and cucumber slices around the avocado. Drizzle everything with dressing. Cover the salad with lemon or lime zest. Lightly sprinkle with freshly ground pepper.

148 Alligator Avocado Snack

INGREDIENTS

1 AVOCADO
JUICE OF ½ LEMON
2 OZ (50G) OF HARD CHEESE
3 PINEAPPLE RINGS
9 OZ (250G) OF SHRIMP
5 SLICES OF PICKLED MUSHROOMS
SALT & PEPPER
1 TBSP OF MAYONNAISE
A SPRIG OF PARSLEY OR CELERY FOR SERVING

PREPARATION

Cut the avocado in half. Remove the pit and sprinkle the pulp with lemon juice. Cut the cheese, pineapple, and avocado pulp into cubes. Add cooked shrimps and sliced mushrooms. Season with salt, pepper, and mayonnaise. Fill the avocado skins with this mixture.

SERVING

Lay out the filled avocado skins on a platter. Decorate the dish with a sprig of parsley or celery.

149 Baked Alligator Avocado Snack

INGREDIENTS

1 AVOCADO
JUICE OF ½ LEMON
2 OZ (50G) OF HARD CHEESE
1 BUNCH OF PARSLEY
7 OZ (200G) OF COOKED SHRIMP
2 PINEAPPLE RINGS
2 RINGS OF CHEESE FOR SERVING
BLACK PEPPER
A SPRIG OF POTHERBS OR A CELERY STALK FOR
SERVING

PREPARATION

Cut the avocado in half. Remove the pulp with a spoon and sprinkle it with lemon juice. Mash the avocado pulp. Add grated cheese, finely chopped parsley, and chopped shrimp. Fill the avocado skins with this mixture and bake at 400°F (200°C) for 20 minutes.

SERVING

Place the filled avocado skins on a serving plate. Put pineapple rings filled with cheese beside the boat. Decorate the dish with a sprig of parsley or dill or a celery stalk.

150 Mermaid Salad

INGREDIENTS

14 OZ (400G) OF SHRIMP
1 WHOLE BAY LEAF
5 PEAS OF ALLSPICE
1 PEAR
½ PINEAPPLE
4 HARDBOILED QUAIL EGGS
1 AVOCADO
3 TBSP OF CREAM
¼ TSP OF CUMIN
1" (2CM) OF GINGER ROOT
1 CLOVE OF GARLIC
LETTUCE LEAVES FOR SERVING
SALT
1 JAR OF BLACK OLIVES

PREPARATION

Boil the shrimp with the bay leaf and allspice for 5 minutes and then peel it. Cut the pear into cubes. Peel the pineapple and cut it into cubes. Boil the quail eggs and cut them in half. Remove the pulp from the avocado and slice it.

Whip the cream. Mix in cumin seeds, grated ginger root, and minced garlic. Mix the pineapple, shrimp, pear, and avocado. Season this mixture with the spiced cream.

SERVING

Cover a plate with lettuce leaves and lay out the dressed salad on top. Decorate half the plate with halved eggs and use black olives on the rest.

151 Quince Turkey Topped with Blue Cheese & Saffron

INGREDIENTS

1 QUINCE
2 TBSP OF CRANBERRIES
17.5 OZ (500G) OF MINCED TURKEY BREAST
1 EGG WHITE
3.5 OZ (100G) OF BLUE CHEESE
2.5 OZ (75G) OF 20% FAT CREAM
A PINCH OF SAFFRON

PREPARATION

Peel the quince and cut it into small cubes. Soak in water until tender. Blend the cranberries and add them.

Season the turkey with salt and pepper. Divide the turkey into 4 flat cakes. In the center of each cake, place a dollop of drained quince and cranberry stuffing. Leave some for serving. Roll the turkey and fruit stuffing up to form meatballs. Cover the meatballs in egg white. Bake the meatballs at 350°F (180°C) for 30 minutes. Mix chopped blue cheese into the cream and warm it over low heat for 1 minute.

SERVING

Place 2 meatballs on a dish. Pour sauce over them and sprinkle with saffron. Garnish the dish with quince.

193

152 Stuffed Quince Covered in Breadcrumbs

INGREDIENTS

1 QUINCE
7 OZ (200G) OF BONELESS, SKINLESS CHICKEN
1 ONION
1 TBSP OF SOUR CREAM
1 TBSP OF MAYONNAISE
SALT & PEPPER
1 TBSP OF BREADCRUMBS
CHOPPED POTHERBS FOR SERVING

PREPARATION

Slice the quince into halves and remove the core and seeds. Scoop out the quince pulp, leaving about ½" (1cm) in the skin. Cut the pulp into cubes. Cut the chicken into cubes of the same size. Chop the onion and lightly fry it. Add quince and continue frying, and then add chicken. Stir everything and remove the pan from heat. Add sour cream, mayonnaise, salt, and pepper to your taste. Put the filling into the quince baskets and sprinkle with finely chopped breadcrumbs. Pour some water on the bottom of the baking pan and bake at 400°F (200°C) for 40 minutes.

SERVING

Lay out the dish on a serving plate. Sprinkle with potherbs of your choice.

153 New Orleans Cotignac Dessert

INGREDIENTS

26.5 OZ (750G) OF QUINCE
14 FL OZ (400 ML) OF WATER
2 FL OZ (65 ML) OF DRY WINE
15 OZ (425G) OF SUGAR
½ LEMON
3.5 OZ (100G) OF CHEESE FOR SERVING

PREPARATION

Wash the quince and cut it into quarters. Remove the core and seeds. Slice what remains and put it in a large saucepan. Fill halfway with water and then add the dry wine. Simmer on low heat until softened. Reduce the contents to a purée, stirring constantly. Put the purée in a clay bowl and let cool. Strain through a sieve.

Boil the water with the sugar and lemon juice until it is reduced to a syrup. Combine the syrup with the quince purée and let simmer for 4 minutes. Let cool and put into silicone baking molds at room temperature for 1 day to harden. Remove from molds with a knife.

SERVING

Lay out on a platter or serving dish with your favorite cheese.

154 Pumpkin Quince Dessert

INGREDIENTS

7 OZ (200G) OF COOKED PUMPKIN PULP
1 QUINCE
2 TBSP OF HONEY
8 WHOLE ALMONDS
1 TBSP OF CREAM
A PINCH OF NUTMEG
SEVERAL GRAPES FOR SERVING

PREPARATION

Slice the pumpkin into cubes. Boil the pumpkin and whole quince for 10 minutes. Strain through a sieve. Peel the quince and remove the seeds. Mix the quince, pumpkin, honey, 4 almonds, and cream in a blender.

SERVING

Lay out the paste in 2 dessert bowls. Decorate with the remaining almonds and sprinkle with nutmeg.

155 Fragrant Quince with Nuts

INGREDIENTS

2 TBSP OF WALNUT KERNELS
2 QUINCE
2 TSP OF BUTTER
2 TBSP OF SUGAR
4 TBSP OF HONEY

PREPARATION

Fry the walnuts without oil. Grind them coarsely in a blender (or chop them with a knife). Peel the quince, remove the core, and cut into slices. Oil a baking pan and tightly pack the quince slices on it. Sprinkle them with sugar. Evenly spread the butter on top of the quince. Bake at 325°F (170°C) for 20 minutes. Drain the juice and mix it with honey.

SERVING

Lay out the quince slices on a large dish. Pour the mixture of honey and juice over it. Sprinkle the dish with nuts.

156 Green Watermelon Cocktail

INGREDIENTS

LEAVES OF LEMON BALM, MINT, & LETTUCE
9 OZ (250G) OF WATERMELON PULP
3.5 FL OZ (100 ML) OF WATER
WATERMELON SLICE & MINT LEAF FOR SERVING

PREPARATION

Put the potherbs, watermelon, and water in a blender and liquefy.

SERVING

Serve the drink in a tall glass. Place the watermelon slice and mint leaf beside the glass on a plate.

157 Watermelon Jelly Dessert

INGREDIENTS

1 WATERMELON
1 OZ (30G) OF GELATIN
A SPRIG OF MINT FOR SERVING
7 FL OZ (200 ML) OF YOUR FAVORITE WINE

PREPARATION

Cut the watermelon in half and remove the pulp with a spoon. Remove the seeds and liquefy in a blender. Add water to the gelatin and combine with the watermelon paste. Fill the empty watermelon halves with the mixture. Freeze and then cut into portions.

SERVING

Place watermelon jelly slices on a large platter and decorate with a sprig of mint.

158 Watermelon Gazpacho

INGREDIENTS

2 CUPS OF WATERMELON PULP
2 FL OZ (50 ML) OF CRANBERRY JUICE
1 TBSP OF CHOPPED CUCUMBER
1 TBSP OF CHOPPED RED BELL PEPPER
1 TSP OF FINELY CHOPPED RED ONION
2 TBSP OF CHOPPED CELERY
1 TBSP OF LIME OR LEMON JUICE
½ TSP OF CHOPPED JALAPEÑO
1 TBSP OF WINE VINEGAR
1 TSP OF PARSLEY

PREPARATION

Mix the watermelon pulp and cranberry juice in a blender. Strain this mixture through a sieve. Add cucumber, bell pepper, onion, celery, lime or lemon juice, watermelon cubes, jalapeño, and vinegar. Stir everything and refrigerate.

SERVING

Pour the gazpacho into 2 tall glasses. Serve the drink with vegetables cut into strips.

159 Watermelon Ice Drink

INGREDIENTS

9 OZ (250G) OF WATERMELON PULP
2 TBSP OF SUGAR
4 TBSP OF LIME JUICE
3.5 FL OZ (100 ML) OF TEQUILA
1 LIME
ICE CUBES FOR SERVING

PREPARATION

Mix the watermelon pulp, sugar, lime juice, and tequila in a blender and strain it through a sieve. Refrigerate until ready to serve. Cut the lime into wedges for serving.

SERVING

Fill a pitcher with ice cubes and add the drink. Put limes wedges on the rims of cocktail glasses and pour the drink.

160 Watermelon Slash

INGREDIENTS

6 ICE CUBES
2 CUPS OF WATERMELON PULP
1 TSP OF HONEY
2 RINGS OF LIME OR LEMON
2 SPRIGS OF MINT FOR SERVING

PREPARATION

Crush the ice in a blender with the watermelon pulp. Add honey and mix gently.

SERVING

Pour the mix into 2 cocktail glasses. Serve with a straw. Decorate the glasses with lemon and mint.

161 Beef in a Banana Blanket

INGREDIENTS

1 LB (½ KG) OF BEEF
SALT
2 RIPE BANANAS
2 KIWI FRUIT
3.5 OZ (100G) OF ANY VARIETY OF CHEESE
1 CUCUMBER
1 TOMATO
PARSLEY
LEMON JUICE FOR SERVING

PREPARATION

Cut the beef into thin slices and season with salt. Peel bananas and kiwi and cut them into thin slices.

Cover a baking pan with foil and lay the beef on top. Put the kiwi and banana slices on the beef. Grate the cheese and sprinkle it on the bananas. Bake at 400°F (200°C) for 60 minutes. Cut the cucumber and tomatoes into slices for serving.

SERVING

Lay out the meat and fruit slices on plates. Place the cucumber and tomatoes slices beside the meat. Decorate the dish with a sprig of parsley. Pour lemon juice over the dish.

162 Chocolate Banana Crisps

INGREDIENTS

9 OZ (250G) OF OAT FLAKES
7 OZ (200G) OF FLOUR   .
3.5 OZ (100G) OF BUTTER
2.5 OZ (75G) OF SUGAR
4 SCOOPS OF VANILLA OR CHOCOLATE ICE CREAM
2 SPRIGS OF MINT FOR SERVING

FILLING:
5 RIPE BANANAS
2 TBSP OF LEMON JUICE
1 TSP OF LEMON ZEST
2 TBSP OF BROWN SUGAR
3.5 OZ (100G) OF GRATED CHOCOLATE

PREPARATION

Mix the oat flakes, flour, butter and sugar into a paste and divide it into 2 equal portions. Put 1 portion in a 10" (24cm) baking dish. Peel the bananas and cut them into slices. Mix with lemon juice, lemon zest, and brown sugar. Pour it over the oat paste layer. Sprinkle with grated chocolate. Spread the second portion of oat paste on top of the bananas. Bake at 400°F (200°C) for 25 minutes.

SERVING

Cut the crisps into portions. Lay out on a plate with ice cream beside each. Decorate the dish with a sprig of mint.

163 Banana Parfait

INGREDIENTS

3 BANANAS
10 OZ (300G) OF COTTAGE CHEESE
½ CUP OF 20% FAT SOUR CREAM
3 TBSP OF POWDERED SUGAR
1 TSP OF GROUND CINNAMON
2 TBSP OF SWEETENED CONDENSED MILK
CHOCOLATE CHIPS FOR SERVING

PREPARATION

Peel and chop the bananas. Mix them with the cottage cheese, cream, powdered sugar, and cinnamon in a blender. Pour this mixture into molds and refrigerate.

SERVING

Lay out the contents of the molds on a serving plate. Pour condensed milk over everything. Decorate the banana parfait with chocolate chips.

164 Chocolate Peanut Banana Skewers

INGREDIENTS

2 BANANAS
3.5 OZ (100G) OF DARK CHOCOLATE
1 CUP OF ROASTED CHOPPED PEANUTS
A SPRIG OF MINT FOR SERVING

PREPARATION

Peel each banana and cut into 4 pieces. Melt the chocolate in a pot over low heat. Stick a wooden skewer into each banana slice and dip in melted chocolate. Roll in chopped peanuts. Lay the bananas on parchment paper, and refrigerate to harden.

SERVING

Lay out the banana skewers on a large rectangular dish. Decorate the dish with a sprig of mint.

165 No Bake Banana & Apple Cheesecake

INGREDIENTS

1 TBSP OF GELATIN
1 CUP OF RYE BREADCRUMBS
½ CUP OF DRIED APRICOTS
½ CUP OF DRIED APPLES
½ CUP OF RAISINS
1 TSP OF LIQUID HONEY
1 APPLE
2 LARGE BANANAS
7 OZ (200G) OF CHEESE
3.5 FL OZ (100 ML) OF MILK
3.5 OZ (100G) OF SUGAR
CINNAMON TO YOUR TASTE

PREPARATION

Soak the gelatin in water, heat, and let cool. Mix the breadcrumbs, dried fruit, and honey in a blender. Grease the walls of a cake mold and pour in the dried fruit mix as a base layer. Peel the apple and bananas and cut into thin slices, leaving some banana aside for serving. Mix the bananas, cottage cheese, milk, sugar, and cinnamon in a blender. Pour the cooled gelatin into this mixture. Lay out the apple slices on the dried fruit layer in the mold. Pour the gelatin and cheese into the mold. Refrigerate for 3-4 hours.

SERVING

Put the cheesecake on a large platter and slice it. Decorate each piece with a banana slice.

166 Champagne Foreplay

INGREDIENTS

2 APPLES
1 MANGO
1 BUNCH OF PURPLE OR PINK GRAPES
1 SMALL PINEAPPLE
1 ORANGE
4 TANGERINES
1 BANANA
2 KIWI
JUICE OF 1 ORANGE
10 FL OZ (300 ML) OF YOUR FAVORITE CHAMPAGNE
FOR SERVING
SEEDS OF 1 SMALL POMEGRANATE

PREPARATION

Peel the apples and mango, cutting them into slices. Cut the grapes in half and remove the seeds. Peel the pineapple and cut it into cubes. Separate the orange and tangerines into segments. Cut the banana and kiwi into slices. Mix all the fruit thoroughly and add the orange juice. Split the salad into 2 dessert bowls.

SERVING

Right before serving, pour your favorite sparkling champagne over the salad and sprinkle it with pomegranate seeds.

167 Grapes & Blue Cheese Salad

INGREDIENTS

1 PEAR
3.5 OZ (100G) OF BLUE CHEESE
2 OZ (50G) OF GRAPES
1 TBSP OF OLIVE OIL
1 TBSP OF BALSAMIC VINEGAR
1 TBSP OF WALNUTS
A SPRIG OF THYME FOR SERVING
A FEW LEAVES OF ARUGULA

PREPARATION

Slice the pear. Cut the cheese into cubes.

SERVING

Lay out the pear and cheese slices on a plate. Place grapes between them. Drizzle everything with olive oil and vinegar. Sprinkle the salad with roasted walnuts. Decorate with thyme and arugula.

168 Delightful Fruit Baskets

INGREDIENTS

5 OZ (150G) OF PINK GRAPES
1 PINK GRAPEFRUIT
3.5 OZ (100G) OF PINEAPPLE
1 BANANA
2 TANGERINES
2 SPRIGS OF MINT FOR SERVING

SAUCE:
2 OZ (50G) OF SOUR CREAM
2 OZ (50G) OF YOGURT
1 ORANGE
SUGAR
A FEW SPRIGS OF LEMON BALM

PREPARATION

Remove the seeds from the grapes. Peel the grapefruit, sep-
arating the pulp from the film and cut it into cubes. Cut the
pineapple into cubes and slice the banana into rings. Divide
the tangerines into slices. Cut the orange in half and juice
it, setting the empty peels aside for serving.

To prepare the sauce: combine sour cream, yogurt, orange
juice, sugar and chopped lemon balm.

SERVING

Serve the salad inside the orange peels. Decorate with mint.

169 Grape Parade

INGREDIENTS

4 PEACHES
2 OZ (50G) OF SUGAR
2 OZ (50G) OF BUTTER
3.5 OZ (100G) OF ROQUEFORT CHEESE
GROUND CINNAMON TO TASTE
17.5 OZ (500G) OF DARK GRAPES
10 OZ (300G) OF FIGS

PREPARATION

Cut the peaches in half and remove the pits. Sprinkle them with sugar and then fry them in butter, cut side down. Fill the empty pits with cheese and sprinkle them with cinnamon.

SERVING

Lay out the peaches on plates with cheese, grapes, and figs on a large dish.

170 Banquet Grape Dessert

INGREDIENTS

2 KIWI FRUITS
1 APPLE
1 ORANGE
1 BANANA
1 TBSP OF POPPY SEEDS
½ CUP OF GRAPES
A FEW SPRIGS OF MINT FOR SERVING

PREPARATION

Peel the kiwi, apple, and orange, and cut them into cubes. Mix the banana and poppy seeds with a small about of water in a blender to make banana sauce.

SERVING

Pour a layer of banana sauce into a glass. Add a layer of apples and grapes, followed by more sauce. Top that with a layer of kiwi and orange, also covering them with sauce. Decorate with a sprig of mint.

171 Blancmange with Strawberry

INGREDIENTS

1 TBSP OF GELATIN
1 CUP OF WATER
17.5 OZ (500G) OF SOUR CREAM
SUGAR
VANILLA
STRAWBERRIES
SEVERAL SPRIGS OF MINT
COCONUT FLAKES FOR SERVING

PREPARATION

Soak the gelatin in cold water, leaving it to swell for 40 minutes. Beat the sour cream with sugar and vanilla. Warm the gelatin and add it to the sour cream. Cut the strawberries in half and put them into glasses or dessert bowls. Pour the sour cream with gelatin mixture over the strawberries. After 3-4 hours when the gelatin is nearly hardened, put a strawberry into each glass to decorate the dish.

SERVING

Serve the dish in glasses decorated with a sprig of mint. Sprinkle the jelly with coconut flakes.

172 Strawberry Chili Sorbet

INGREDIENTS

1 BOTTLE OF DRY RED WINE
5 OZ (150G) OF POWDERED SUGAR
ZEST OF 2 ORANGES
5 WHOLE CLOVES
10 PEAS OF HOT PEPPER
1LB (½KG) OF STRAWBERRIES
SEVERAL MINT LEAVES FOR SERVING

PREPARATION

Combine wine, powdered sugar, orange zest, cloves, and pepper in a saucepan. Cook over low heat until the liquid is reduced to half. Strain the water and put the contents in a mold. Let cool and freeze, occasionally stirring for an even freeze.

SERVING

Put coarsely chopped strawberries into 2 tall glasses or deep plates. Sprinkle with powdered sugar through a sieve. Top the strawberries with sorbet balls and dessert spoons, and decorate the dish with mint leaves.

173 Strawberry Carpaccio

INGREDIENTS

17.5 OZ (500G) OF FRESH LARGE STRAWBERRIES
5 TBSP OF BROWN OR REGULAR SUGAR
2.5 FL OZ (70 ML) OF BALSAMIC VINEGAR
A HANDFUL OF FRESH MINT LEAVES
A PINCH OF VANILLA
2 TBSP OF POWDERED SUGAR
2 SPRIGS OF MINT FOR SERVING

PREPARATION

Cut the strawberries into very thin slices with a sharp knife.

To prepare the dressing, mix sugar with balsamic vinegar. Add 5 tablespoons of water and reduce to a thick, viscous mass.

SERVING

Lay out the strawberries on 2 dishes in a shape of a fan (from the center of the plate to its edges). Sprinkle with chopped mint and pour it over with balsamic sauce. Add a pinch of vanilla to powdered sugar and sprinkle the strawberry carpaccio through a sieve with it. Place a sprig of mint in the center of the composition.

174 Strawberry & Vanilla Pudding with Chia Seeds

INGREDIENTS

7 OZ (200G) OF FRESH STRAWBERRIES
½ CUP OF ALMOND MILK
2 TSP OF PURE VANILLA EXTRACT
2 TBSP OF CHIA SEEDS
2 STRAWBERRIES FOR SERVING

PREPARATION

Mix strawberries, almond milk and vanilla extract in a blender. Pour this mixture over the chia seeds. Let sit for 3 minutes and mix again. Refrigerate for 30 minutes or until thickened. Stir again before serving.

SERVING

Put the pudding into individual dessert bowls. Decorate each bowl with a whole strawberry.

175 Strawberry Philadelphia Dessert

INGREDIENTS

17.5 OZ (500G) OF FRESH STRAWBERRIES
7 OZ (200G) OF PHILADELPHIA CREAM CHEESE
½ CUP OF POWDERED SUGAR
2 TBSP OF MILK
CHOCOLATE CRUMBS FOR SERVING

PREPARATION

Remove the stems from the strawberries and hollow them out from the base. Whip the cream cheese, powdered sugar, and milk into an airy cream. Fill this cream inside each hollowed out strawberry using a pastry bag.

SERVING

Lay out the strawberries on a large serving dish. Sprinkle them with chocolate crumbs.

176 ManMak Salad

INGREDIENTS

1 RADICCHIO
5 OZ (150G) OF WALNUTS
2 CLOVES OF GARLIC
3 TBSP OF OLIVE OIL
3 TBSP OF MACADAMIA OIL
3 TBSP OF LEMON JUICE
1 MANGO
1 AVOCADO
YOUR FAVORITE SPICES TO TASTE
1 TBSP OF GREEN BASIL LEAVES
1 TBSP OF WATERCRESS
20 COOKED & PEELED SHRIMP
SEVERAL BASIL LEAVES FOR SERVING

PREPARATION

Collect the pink leaves from the radicchio. Fry lightly chopped walnuts and garlic in olive and macadamia oil for 5 minutes. After 30 seconds, remove from heat and add lemon juice, mango, and avocado slices. Season everything with your favorite spices.

SERVING

Lay out radicchio leaves, basil, and watercress on a large platter. Top with shrimp. Pour mango, macadamia, and avocado sauce over everything. Decorate the dish with basil leaves.

177 Mango, Avocado, & Trout Salad

INGREDIENTS

1 MANGO
1 AVOCADO
7 OZ (200G) OF SALTED TROUT
10 OZ (300G) OF SALAD GREENS OF YOUR CHOICE
SALT & PEPPER

SAUCE:
4 TBSP OF OLIVE OIL
3 TBSP OF WHOLEGRAIN MUSTARD
2 TSP OF LEMON JUICE

PREPARATION

Peel the mango and avocado and cut them into thin slices. Cut the trout into small pieces. Combine the trout with the mango, avocado, and salad greens. To prepare the sauce: mix olive oil, mustard, and lemon juice.

SERVING

Lay out the salad on a plate and cover it with the sauce. Add salt and pepper to your taste.

178 Crystal Salad

INGREDIENTS

4 OZ (120G) OF RICE NOODLES
3 LEEKS
1 MANGO
1 TSP OF CHOPPED JALAPEÑO
17.5 OZ (500G) OF COOKED & PEELED SHRIMP
1 TBSP OF CHOPPED BASIL

DRESSING:
⅓ CUP OF RICE VINEGAR
1 TSP OF SALT
2 TBSP OF SUGAR

PREPARATION

Pour boiling water over the rice noodles and let sit for 8 minutes. Drain and rinse with cold water. Cut the leek into rings, slice the mango, and chop the jalapeño. Mix the mango, shrimp, leek, jalapeño, and basil together. Blend vinegar with salt and sugar into a sauce. Pour half of the sauce over the rice and half as a dressing for the salad.

SERVING

Put the salad in the bottom of a salad bowl. Put the rice noodles on top of the salad, and the shrimp mixture on top of the rice noodles.

179 Mango Parma Salad

INGREDIENTS

1 HEAD OF ROMAINE LETTUCE
1 BUNCH OF ARUGULA
1 MANGO
8 CHERRY TOMATOES
8 PIECES OF MINI MOZZARELLA CHEESE
2 TSP OF PESTO SAUCE
3 OZ (80G) OF PARMA HAM

DRESSING:
2 TBSP OF OLIVE OIL
2 TBSP OF BALSAMIC VINEGAR
1 TSP OF MUSTARD
SEA SALT & BLACK PEPPER

PREPARATION

Wash and dry the romaine lettuce and arugula. Peel the mango and cut it into cubes. Wrap slices of ham around the mango cubes to form rolls and fasten with a toothpick. Cut the cherry tomatoes in half and arrange them on wooden skewers, alternating with mini mozzarella balls. Coat these kebabs with pesto sauce.

To prepare the dressing: mix olive oil, balsamic vinegar, mustard, pepper, and salt. Drizzle onto lettuce and arugula.

SERVING

Arrange the salad in the center of a large serving plate. Place the mango and Parma ham rolls on top. Place 2 kebabs on either edge of the plate.

180 Soft Mango Pudding Soufflé

INGREDIENTS

½ CUP OF ORANGE JUICE
1 TBSP OF LIME JUICE
2 TSP OF INSTANT GELATIN
1 MANGO
½ CUP OF SOUR CREAM
½ CUP OF MILK
⅓ CUP OF SUGAR
2 TBSP OF RUM
1 TBSP OF BRANDY
2 COCKTAIL CHERRIES
2 SPRIGS OF MINT FOR SERVING

PREPARATION

Pour the juices and gelatin into a saucepan. Simmer over low heat until the gelatin is completely dissolved. Cut the mango into slices, leaving several slices aside for serving. Whip the mango, sour cream, milk, sugar, rum, and brandy in a blender. Stir it into the gelatin mixture.

Pour the mixture into portioned dessert bowls and freeze for 2-3 hours. Add mango slices to the semi-frozen soufflé bowls. Continue freezing for another 2-3 hours before serving.

SERVING

Remove the frozen soufflés from the freezer. Decorate with cherries and mint.

222

181 Ginger Beauty Salad

INGREDIENTS

17.5 OZ (500G) OF COUSCOUS
10 OZ (300G) OF DATES
7 OZ (200G) OF DRIED TOMATOES
1 RED ONION
1 CUCUMBER
JUICE OF 2 LEMONS
3.5 FL OZ (100 ML) OF OLIVE OIL
SALT & PEPPER
1 BUNCH OF CILANTRO

PREPARATION

Cook the couscous in water. Cut the dates, dried tomatoes, onion, and cucumber into chunks and add them to the couscous. Mix the lemon juice with the olive oil. Season the salad with salt and pepper. Stir it thoroughly.

SERVING

Place the salad on a large dish. Sprinkle the dish with chopped cilantro.

182 Bacon Wrapped Banquet Dates

INGREDIENTS

10 DATES
7 OZ (200G) OF BLUE CHEESE
10 ROASTED ALMONDS
10 SLICES OF BACON
10 LEAVES OF ARUGULA
BALSAMIC VINEGAR TO TASTE

PREPARATION

Remove the pits from the dates and replace them with chopped blue cheese and almonds. Wrap each date in bacon and fasten the roll with a toothpick. Bake the date rolls at 325°F (170°C) until the bacon turns brown.

SERVING

Arrange banquet spoons with single leaves of arugula on a large dish. Place a date wrap on each leaf. Sprinkle with balsamic vinegar. If you do not have banquet spoons, you can use lettuce leaves instead.

183 Date Snack Balls

INGREDIENTS

1 CUP OF ROASTED ALMONDS
1 ½ CUPS OF DRIED DATES
2 TBSP OF PEANUT BUTTER
4 TBSP OF SESAME SEEDS
1 TSP OF CINNAMON
A PINCH OF SEA SALT

PREPARATION

Grind the almonds in a blender, leaving several whole ones aside for serving. Separately grind the dates in a blender. Mix both pastes and the peanut butter together to form balls. Mix the sesame seeds, cinnamon, and salt and sprinkle the date balls with this mixture. Put the balls into a glass jar and refrigerate until ready to serve.

SERVING

Arrange the date balls on a rectangular plate. Decorate with whole almonds.

184 Date Cakes

INGREDIENTS

7 OZ (200G) OF HAZELNUTS
7 OZ (200G) OF PITTED DATES
3.5 OZ (100G) OF COCOA
2 FL OZ (50 ML) OF MAPLE SYRUP
2 BANANAS
1 OZ (25G) OF POWDERED SUGAR
SEVERAL SPRIGS OF MINT FOR SERVING

PREPARATION

Crush the hazelnuts in a blender. Add dates, half the cocoa, and half the maple syrup and blend into a paste. Roll the paste out into a ½" (1.5cm) thick flat cake. Use a round drinking glass to cut out circles from the cake. Mix banana, the remaining cocoa, and the remaining maple syrup in a blender to make cream. Spread this cream flat between two round cakes.

SERVING

Lay out 2 date cakes per plate. Sprinkle them with powdered sugar. Decorate the dish with a sprig of mint.

185 Palm Dessert

INGREDIENTS

10 OZ (300G) OF DATES
7 OZ (200G) OF ALMONDS
1 COCONUT
10 FL OZ (300 ML) OF EGG LIQUEUR OR MULLED
WINE FOR SERVING

PREPARATION

Finely chop the dates and blanche the almonds. Split the coconut in half, leaving the meat intact. Fill the coconut halves with the date and almond mixture.

SERVING

Serve the coconut halves with egg liqueur or mulled wine.

Section VI: Chocolate

In the 7th century B.C. the ancient Mayans grew cacao beans and cooked them into a bitter drink called chocolatl. It gave them great physical strength and wisdom for life. Europeans didn't learn about chocolate until the 1520's when conquistador Hernan Cortes brought the drink home from his travels with the Aztecs. Chocolatl was prepared using cocoa liquor, honey, and vanilla.

From the Middle Ages to the end of the 19th century, chocolate was only known as a drink. It was not until the 20th century that it became popular throughout the world. Previously, the price of sugar and cocoa had been very high, but a sharp decrease meant many more people could afford it. Today, this dessert of kings is available to everyone.

Thanks to its magnesium content, chocolate improves the mood and energizes the body. Chocolate contains anti-oxidants which help keep us feeling young and beautiful.

Cocoa powder contains phenylethylamine, which stimulates the love center of the brain. It aids in the development of serotonin, the happiness hormone, and helps create positive feelings and a state of mild euphoria. However, it is worth remembering that only bitter, dark chocolate has these properties. This magical food also contains theobromine which gently stimulates the nervous and cardiovascular systems. It is said the French consume 36 thousand tons of chocolate during the holidays, four times the weight of the Eiffel Tower!

You can easily combine chocolate with coffee. Caffeine stimulates the central nervous system, contributing to heightened sexual arousal. A piece of dark chocolate will add endorphins to your hormones and is known to enhance the attraction between two lovers. You can feed each other with fruits dipped in melted chocolate. Use melted chocolate to draw something on your partner's body and then lick it off! All of these combined can create magic and wonder between any couple.

186 Chocolate Risotto

INGREDIENTS

6 FL OZ (180 ML) OF MILK
2 OZ (60G) OF RICE
5 OZ (150G) OF DARK CHOCOLATE
1 TSP OF BUTTER
A HANDFUL OF ANY BERRIES FOR SERVING

PREPARATION

Combine the milk and rice. Bring the mixture to a boil and add the chocolate. Simmer over low heat for 20 minutes, stirring occasionally. Stir in butter and remove from heat.

SERVING

Arrange the risotto on a serving plate. Decorate with berries of your choice.

187 Pear in Chocolate

INGREDIENTS

2 FL OZ (60 ML) OF DRY WINE
1.5 FL OZ (40 ML) OF SWEET WINE
CINNAMON, STAR ANISE, & CLOVES TO TASTE
2 OZ (50G) OF SUGAR
1 PEAR
3.5 OZ (100G) OF DARK CHOCOLATE
2 TBSP OF MILK

PREPARATION

Mix wine with spices and sugar and bring it to a boil. Slice the pear and remove the seeds. Add the pear slices to the wine. Simmer over very low heat for 40 minutes. Melt the chocolate over low heat in the milk.

SERVING

Pour a layer of melted chocolate on the bottom of the dish. Top it with pears and add more melted chocolate. Make small chocolate droplets from chocolate sauce around the pear.

188 Chocolate Velvet

INGREDIENTS

5 OZ (150G) OF DARK CHOCOLATE
3.5 OZ (100G) OF BUTTER
3.5 OZ (100G) OF WHITE CHOCOLATE
2 EGGS
1 TBSP OF SUGAR
1 FL OZ (30 ML) OF CHERRY BRANDY OR SWEET RED
WINE
2 COCKTAIL CHERRIES
CHOPPED NUTS OF ANY VARIETY FOR SERVING

PREPARATION

Melt the dark chocolate with 2 oz (70g) of butter. Melt the white chocolate in the remaining butter, stirring continuously. Separate the egg whites from the yolks. Beat the whites with the sugar to form stable peaks. Add the yolks and beat once again. Slowly add 1 tbsp of the egg mixture to the melted white chocolate. Add cherry brandy or sweet red wine to the dark chocolate. Gradually pour the rest of the egg mixture into the white chocolate. Stir everything gently.

SERVING

Pour the dark chocolate mixture into dessert bowls or martini glasses. Make a spiral of white chocolate mixture on the surface of the dark chocolate using a pastry bag. Refrigerate for 2-3 hours. Decorate the dish with cocktail cherries and chopped nuts.

189 Chocolate Iceberg

INGREDIENTS

2 OZ (50G) OF DARK CHOCOLATE
14 FL OZ (400 ML) OF ANY FRUIT JUICE OR DRY
WHITE WINE
3.5 OZ (100G) OF ICE CREAM

PREPARATION

Grate the chocolate into flakes. Pour half the juice or dry white wine in a tall glass or dessert bowl. Top it with a scoop of ice cream.

SERVING

Generously sprinkle the ice cream with chocolate flakes. Insert a cocktail straw and enjoy.

190 Tropical Chocolate Dessert

INGREDIENTS

2 RIPE BANANAS
JUICE OF 1 ORANGE
2 FL OZ (50 ML) OF CREAM
2 TBSP OF SUGAR OR POWDERED SUGAR
3.5 OZ (100G) OF DARK CHOCOLATE
6 CHOCOLATE CHIPS
2 MINT LEAVES FOR SERVING

PREPARATION

Mix the bananas in a blender with the orange juice. Boil for 5 minutes, stirring constantly. Add cream, sugar, and chocolate. Simmer on low heat until the chocolate is completely melted.

SERVING

Pour the mixture into 2 ice cream bowls and refrigerate for 1 hour. Insert 3 chocolate chips into each ice-cream bowl and decorate with a mint leaf.

Section VII: Love Potions, Hot Drinks, & Spicy Teas

Some of these drink recipes have a very ancient history. Others came around not long ago, but they still have the same powerful properties. Some beverages are suitable for both women and men, while some are recommended either for men or women exclusively.

Sbitens are a type of traditional Russian hot winter drink and are an extremely important component of any erotic cuisine. Sbitens are traditionally prepared only with honey, not sugar. The honey is added to the drinks when they are slightly cooled (to 55 degrees Celsius or 130 degrees Fahrenheit). These drinks can be flavored with orange, lemon, or grapefruit zest.

191 Casanova Beverage

INGREDIENTS

3 CUPS OF WATER
1 TSP OF DRIED RASPBERRY
DRIED MARIGOLD & ROSE LEAVES
1 PINCH OF CUMIN
2 TBSP OF BRANDY

PREPARATION

Boil the water and remove from heat. Add all dried herbs and cumin, leaving them to infuse for 25 minutes. Strain the liquid and add brandy, setting the solids aside. The herbal solids can be mixed with honey to make jam.

SERVING

The Casanova beverage should be drunk by men while it is still warm, immediately after straining.

192 "Anise Love" Mulled Wine

INGREDIENTS

1 APPLE
1 ORANGE
1" (2CM) OF FRESH GINGER ROOT
3 STARS OF ANISE
3 WHOLE CLOVES
A PINCH OF CINNAMON
17 FL OZ (500 ML) OF RED WINE
1 TBSP OF LIQUID HONEY
JUICE & ZEST OF ½ LEMON
2 LEMON SLICES
2 CINNAMON STICKS FOR SERVING

PREPARATION

Peel the apple and the orange and cut them into slices. Peel the ginger and grate it. Place fruit, all spices, red wine, honey, lemon zest, and juice in a large saucepan. Simmer over low heat for 5 minutes.

SERVING

Pour this fragrant drink into mulled wine glasses. Decorate with lemon slices and cinnamon sticks.

193 Estonia Cocktail

INGREDIENTS

1 CUP OF WHITE DESSERT WINE
4 WHOLE CLOVES
A PINCH OF NUTMEG & SAFFRON
2 LEMON SLICES FOR SERVING

PREPARATION

Pour the wine in a saucepan. Add the spices and simmer on low heat for 5 minutes. Strain the spiced wine and refrigerate for 1 hour.

SERVING

Lightly wet the rim of a cocktail glass. Pour sugar on a plate and dip the wet rim to coat it in sugar. Pour the chilled cocktail into this glass. Add a lemon slice to the drink.

194 Hot Love Beverage

INGREDIENTS

2 WHOLE CLOVES
CINNAMON
NUTMEG
A PINCH OF TARRAGON
LEMON ZEST
12 FL OZ (350 ML) OF DRY RED WINE
1 TBSP OF BRANDY
1 TBSP OF SUGAR
2 SLICES OF PEELED ORANGE FOR SERVING

PREPARATION

Add spices and lemon zest to dry red wine, and bring it to a boil. Strain the wine, add brandy and sugar.

SERVING

Serve this drink warm with an orange slice in the glass.

195 Sporty Energy Drink

INGREDIENTS

1 TBSP OF SUGAR
7 FL OZ (200 ML) OF DRY GRAPE WINE
2 FL OZ (60 ML) OF GRAPE JUICE
A PINCH OF NUTMEG
A PINCH OF TARRAGON
2 LEMON SLICES FOR SERVING

PREPARATION

Add the sugar to the wine and let it simmer in a saucepan for a few minutes. Remove from heat and add grape juice and spices. Refrigerate until ready to serve.

SERVING

Pour the drink into tall glasses. Decorate the rim of the glass with a lemon slice.

196 Khoshav Spiced Dried Fruit Compote

INGREDIENTS

17.5 OZ (500G) OF DRIED PRUNES
½ LEMON
SUGAR
8.5 FL OZ (250 ML) OF WHITE WINE
1 CINNAMON STICK
A PINCH OF CARDAMOM
2 LEMON SLICES FOR SERVING

PREPARATION

Submerge the prunes in water and let sit for 12 hours. Add lemon slices and simmer in a saucepan for a few minutes. Add sugar, wine, and spices and continue simmering for a few minutes. Let the wine mixture cool and strain through a sieve.

SERVING

Pour the drink into tall glasses. Put a lemon slice on the rim of each glass.

197 Men's Passion Potion

INGREDIENTS

2 FL OZ (50 ML) GINSENG TINCTURE
2 FL OZ (50 ML) PINK RADIOGRAM TINCTURE
2 FL OZ (50 ML) MANCHURIAN ARALIA TINCTURE
2 FL OZ (50 ML) PRICKLY ELEUTHEROCOCCUS TINC-
TURE

PREPARATION

Mix all the tinctures together thoroughly.

HOW TO CONSUME

Men should take 30 drops 3 times a day after meals.

198 Danae Waits for Zeus

INGREDIENTS

1 TSP OF GRATED HORSERADISH
1 TSP OF ANISE SEEDS
½ TSP OF CUMIN
3 CUPS OF WATER
YOUR FAVORITE FRUITS (OPTIONAL)
2 TBSP OF HONEY

PREPARATION

Add the grated horseradish, anise seeds, and cumin to water in a pot. Optionally, you can also include any fruit of your choice. Bring everything to a boil and immediately remove from heat. Let cool to room temperature and add honey. Stir and leave it to infuse for 15 minutes.

HOW TO CONSUME

Drink this beverage hot in small portions several times throughout the day.

199 Spicy Sbiten

INGREDIENTS

1 TSP OF PEPPERMINT
1 TSP OF ST. JOHN'S WORT
1 TSP OF CHAMOMILE
3 GLASSES OF PURIFIED WATER
1 TSP OF GRATED RADISH OR DAIKON
2 TBSP OF VODKA
2 TBSP OF HONEY

PREPARATION

Put all the herbs in water and bring to a boil. Remove from heat and add radish or daikon. Cover with a lid and leave to infuse for 15 minutes. Strain the mixture, and then add vodka and honey. Stir until honey is dissolved.

HOW TO CONSUME

Drink 3.5 oz (100 ml) of this sbiten several times a day for increased energy.

200 Soft Firuza Drink

INGREDIENTS

1 MELON
ICE
1 CUP OF POMEGRANATE JUICE
1 CUP OF GRAPE JUICE
1 CUP OF SPARKLING WATER
2 MELON SLICES FOR SERVING

PREPARATION

Remove the melon pulp from its skin and cut it into small cubes. Crush the ice in a blender.

SERVING

Take 2 tall glasses. Fill ⅓ of the glasses with crushed ice. Pour ½ cup of pomegranate and grape juice into the glasses. Add melon cubes and pour sparkling water to the top of the glasses. Decorate the rims of the glasses with a melon slice.

201 Nut Milk Beverage

INGREDIENTS

10 WALNUT KERNELS
5 FL OZ (150 ML) OF WATER
2 TSP OF HONEY

PREPARATION

Grind the walnuts in a coffee grinder or blender. Add water and leave to infuse for 2 hours. Strain the drink and add honey.

HOW TO CONSUME

Men should drink this beverage in 2 sittings over the course of a meal. The nut milk beverage has a beneficial effect on spermatogenesis.

202 Pine Nut Water

INGREDIENTS

½ CUP OF PINE NUTS
17 FL OZ (500 ML) OF PURIFIED WATER

PREPARATION

Grind pine nuts in a blender or coffee grinder. Add water and leave to infuse overnight.

HOW TO CONSUME

Drink 3.5 fl oz (100 ml) of this tincture every day.

203 Ginseng Tea

INGREDIENTS

1 TBSP OF GINSENG
2 CUPS OF WATER
1 TBSP OF GRATED GINGER ROOT

PREPARATION

Add ginseng to water and bring it to a boil. Add grated ginger root and leave to infuse for 1-2 hours. Strain the mixture.

HOW TO CONSUME

Drink the tea right before a sexual encounter.

204 Wormwood Tea

INGREDIENTS

1 TBSP OF WORMWOOD
2 CUPS OF WATER
1 TBSP OF GRATED GINGER ROOT

PREPARATION

Add wormwood to water and bring it to a boil. Add grated ginger root and leave to infuse for 1-2 hours. Strain the mixture.

HOW TO CONSUME

Drink the tea right before a sexual encounter.

205 Anise Tea

INGREDIENTS

1 TSP OF ANISE SEEDS
1 CUP OF WATER

PREPARATION

Add 1 tsp of anise seeds to boiling water. Leave it to infuse for 10 minutes and then strain the mixture.

HOW TO CONSUME

Drink a cup of this tea several times throughout the day.

206 Herbal Coffee with Lemon Aftertaste

INGREDIENTS

1 TBSP OF GROUND COFFEE
1 TSP OF DRIED OREGANO
½ TSP OF LEMONGRASS LEAVES
2 CUPS OF WATER
SUGAR

PREPARATION

Mix the ground coffee and herbs. Add the mixture to water and simmer over low heat for 1 minute. Remove from heat and leave to infuse for 5 minutes. Strain the mixture and add sugar to your taste.

207 Anise Seed Tea

INGREDIENTS

1 CUP OF HOT WATER
1 TBSP OF ANISE SEEDS
1 TBSP OF HONEY OR BRANDY

PREPARATION

Boil the water and add the anise seeds. Simmer over low heat for 15 minutes and remove from heat. Leave to infuse for 20 minutes. Strain the seeds from the liquid. Add 1 tablespoon of honey and 1 tbsp of brandy. Stir thoroughly.

HOW TO CONSUME

Women should drink 1 tablespoon of warm anise seed tea 3 times a day.

208 Maral Root Drink

INGREDIENTS

3 TBSP OF MARAL ROOT
34 OZ (1 LITER) OF WATER

PREPARATION

Add the maral root to the water and let infuse for 3 hours.
Strain the mixture.

HOW TO CONSUME

Drink 1 tablespoon 3 times a day before meals.

209 Guarana Passion Drink

INGREDIENTS

34 OZ (1 LITER) OF WATER
2 TBSP OF GUARANA SEEDS

PREPARATION

Boil the water. Remove from heat and add the guarana seeds. Leave it to infuse for 10 minutes.

HOW TO CONSUME

Drink this beverage throughout the day before a romantic evening.

Conclusion

Armed with the knowledge contained in this cookbook, you'll be able to craft affordable dishes that will create an atmosphere of love, harmony, and sexual celebration.

It has long been believed that the most honorable of all occupations are teaching, healing, and nurturing. Chefs in France are considered equal to great artists. The ability to cook meals for erotic purposes is even greater still. Use the recipes offered here, but also use your imagination to create your own original culinary delights for your partner! Approach cooking an erotic meal with a joyful and confident mood, as an easy and fun process. You will create an unforgettable experience for both the stomach and loins.

Remember, the more varied the range of dishes you eat, the more likely that your body will receive all the vitamins and minerals needed to increase sexual endurance.

Finally, this book should not be taken as a complete guide. My goal was to add some spice, some romance, and something special you may have lost back to your daily life. In addition to the added health and pleasure the foods here offer, you will gain valuable cooking skills you can use to surprise your loved one and make yourself feel like an artist. Bon appétit!

Acknowledgements

Thank you to all the people who helped to make this book possible. It's truly a collective work. Without help from others, these recipes would have stayed forever among only my family and close friends in Ukraine. I am very grateful for the opportunity to share them with other nations and cultures.

I would especially like to thank Emma Taylor and Andrea L. Purvis, two people who dedicated their care and cooking skills to make this book stand out. In my humble opinion, Andrea makes the best spiced ginger cookies in the world, and I could learn a few things from her. My lovely daughter, Anastasia Petrenko, and her partner, Grego-ry Diehl, used their significant artistic talent, writing, and voices to polish and publish the final version you now get to enjoy. I am very fortunate to have their help to bring my dream to reality.

I believe that everyone who uses my recipes in the right mood will have no regrets and see undeniable results. I hope they become favorites in your kitchen and will help bring you closer to the people you care about.

Bibliography

Alan R. Hirsch, M.D., F.A.C.P., and Jason J. Gruss (2014). *Human Male Sexual Response to Olfactory Stimuli | The American Academy of Neurological and Orthopaedic Surgeons.* [online] Available at: http://aanos.org/human-male-sexual-response-to-olfactory-stimuli/ [Accessed 3 Jan. 2017].

Xiao Deng, Qianghong Pu, Erhao Wang, and Chao Yu (2016). *Celery extract inhibits mouse CYP2A5 and human CYP2A6 activities via different mechanisms | Institute of Life Sciences, Chongqing Medical University, Chongqing 400016, P.R. China.* [online] Available at: https://www.spandidos-publications.com/ol/12/6/5309/download [Accessed 3 Jan. 2017].

John P. Melnyk, Massimo F. Marcone (2011). *Aphrodisiacs from Plant and Animal Sources – A Review of Current Scientific Literature. Food Research International.* [online] Available at: http://www.sciencedirect.com/science/article/pii/S0963996911001451/ [Accessed 3 Jan. 2017].

Steels, E., Rao, A. and Vitetta, L. (2011). *Physiological Aspects of Male Libido Enhanced by Standardized Trigonella foenum-graecum Extract and Mineral Formulation.* [online] Wiley Online Library. Available at: http://onlinelibrary.wiley.com/doi/10.1002/ptr.3360/full [Accessed 3 Jan. 2017].

Forest, C., Padma-Nathan, H. and Liker, H. (2007). *Efficacy and safety of pomegranate juice on improvement of erectile dysfunction in male patients with mild to moderate erectile dysfunction: a randomized, placebo-controlled, double-blind, crossover study.* [online] *International Journal of Impotence Research.* Available at: http://www.nature.com/ijir/journal/v19/n6/abs/3901570a.html [Accessed 3 Jan. 2017].

Index

Ginkgo Biloba, xv
ginseng, ix, xii, xv, 244, 250
glutamic acid, 48, 50
grape, x, 91, 160, 171, 176, 196, 208, 209, 210, 211, 212
grape juice, 175, 176, 242, 247
grapefruit, 29, 43, 44, 210, 237
Greece, ix, 1, 2, 5, 38, 42, 116
guarana, 256
hake, 47, 107
herbs, xiii, 107, 238, 246, 253
herring, iv, 49, 50, 67, 68, 69
Hippocampus Coronatus, xii
honey, xiii, xvi, 6, 13, 19, 20, 36, 42, 43, 44, 79, 122, 133, 152,
    161, 171, 174, 176, 180, 184, 196, 197, 202, 207, 229, 237,
    238, 239, 245, 246, 248, 254
horseradish, 23, 55, 67, 99, 101, 102, 245
hot pepper, 96, 99, 162, 214
hot sauce, 96
ice cream, 172
Impaza, xii
India, xiii, 179
iodine, 2, 47, 50, 52, 114, 115, 116, 117, 150, 179
iron, 2, 3, 7, 52, 113, 115, 117, 150, 174, 175, 179, 181
Italy, ii, xiii, 14, 26, 29, 36, 37, 72
jalapeño, 200, 220
Japan, ii, x, 27, 30, 146, 179
Kabul sauce, 65, 66
kale, 119
kelp, vii, 113, 117, 143, 144, 145, 146, 147
ketchup, 54, 130, 134
kiwi, 184, 203, 208, 212
kohlrabi, 5, 36
kumquat, 178
ladyfingers, 187
leek, 6, 21, 56, 97, 220
lemon juice, 10, 11, 20, 21, 27, 30, 31, 32, 41, 42, 54, 56, 61,
    71, 73, 74, 77, 79, 81, 82, 84, 86, 89, 90, 92, 93, 94, 95, 107,
    108, 119, 120, 123, 125, 137, 138, 142, 144, 151, 152, 155,
    159, 160, 162, 171, 182, 183, 185, 188, 189, 190, 191, 195,
    200, 203, 204, 218, 219, 223
lemon zest, 11, 27, 56, 62, 71, 73, 152, 204, 239, 241

About the Author

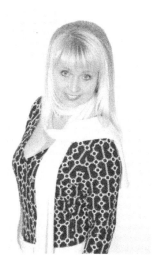

Olga Petrenko grew up in Ukraine, where she learned to appreciate traditional Eastern European hospitality and homemaking. As an adult, she studied the chemistry of foods, both local and foreign, for their unique effects on the human body and mind. Combining her food science studies with her love for helping others achieve greater intimacy, she poured the next 10 years of her life into creating the recipes contained in her first book, *Intimacy On The Plate*. She enjoys a fantastic love life with her husband of 35 years and maintains a diverse herbal garden at home.

Come see where unique and meaningful ideas live.

Like Identity Publications on
Facebook.com/identitypublications

Follow Identity Publications on
Twitter.com/identitypublic

Subscribe to Identity Publications on
Youtube.com/c/identitypublications

Find out more about our publishing approach at
IdentityPublications.com

Made in United States
Orlando, FL
21 January 2023

28883259R00189